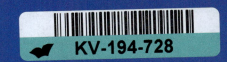

Contents

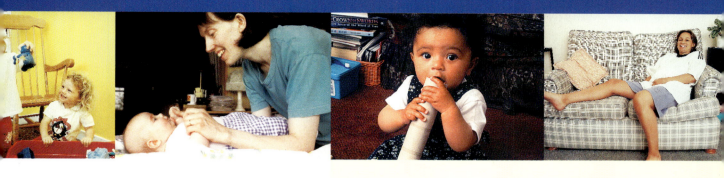

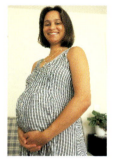
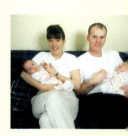

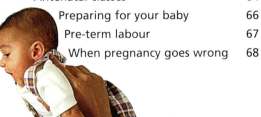

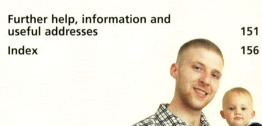

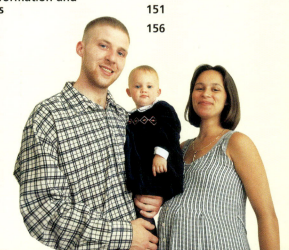

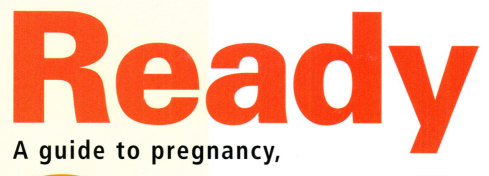

Ready Steady Baby!

A guide to pregnancy, birth and early parenthood

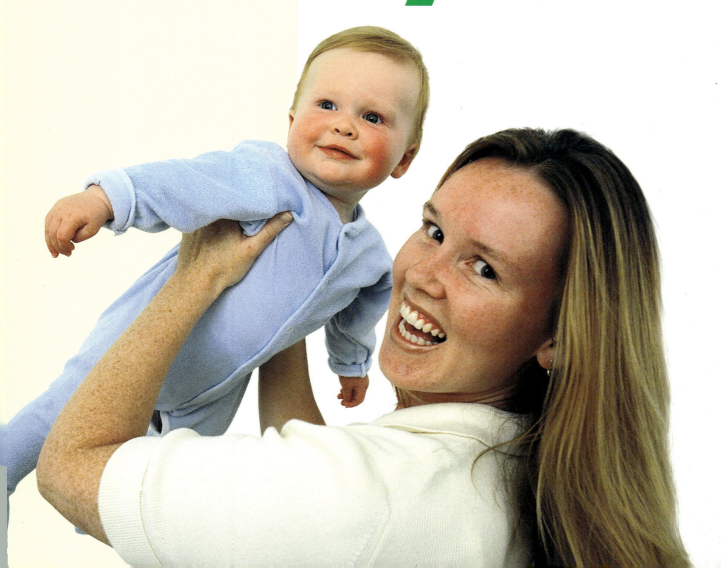

Acknowledgements

This book reflects many discussions, suggestions and comments made by health professionals, professional bodies, lay and voluntary organisations, and parents. Health Scotland would like to thank all of those who contributed in any way to the development of this project, for so willingly giving their time, and sharing their expertise and experience.

Special thanks to the task group responsible for working on this project, especially Gill Allan, Linda Bryce, Sally Callaghan, Nadine Edwards, Kirsty Foster, Leslie Marr, Agnes McGowan, Jean Muir, Jenny Warren, Linda Wolfson and Riny Wondergem. Dr Sheila Lawson, Dr Angus Ford and Clare Keenan also provided valuable input and support.

Particular thanks to all the parents who gave permission for us to take and use photographs of themselves and their children.

This book was produced with the support of Borders Community Health Services NHS Trust, Dundee Teaching Hospital (Ninewells), Lanarkshire Health Board, Law Hospital NHS Trust, Lothian Health, Simpson Memorial Maternity Pavilion, West Lothian and Yorkhill NHS Trusts.

Published by Health Scotland.

Edinburgh Office: Woodburn House, Canaan Lane, Edinburgh EH10 4SG
Glasgow Office: Clifton House, Clifton Place, Glasgow G3 7LS

© NHS Health Scotland, 1998,1999, 2002, 2003, 2004.

First published 1998
Second edition 1999
Revised 2002, 2003, 2004

ISBN: 1-84485-239-3

www.healthscotland.com

Original text: Heather Welford

Design: Design Links, Edinburgh/Glasgow

Photography: Iain Stewart. Pages 78, 79, 80, 82 and 84: Collections / Anthea Sieveking — thanks to Janet Balaskas and the Active Birth Movement for their part in arranging these pictures.

Printed by Acorn Web

Every effort has been made to ensure that this publication is as up to date and accurate as possible. However, new medical research can sometimes mean that information about pregnancy and childbirth, and recommendations for childcare change very quickly. Changes and alterations will be made at the next reprint to reflect any new information, and significant changes in recommendations will be made at once to doctors, midwives and health visitors.

While the book represents the consensus of good practice, please remember that different circumstances and clinical judgement may mean that you have slightly different patterns of care.

If you have any doubts, worries or fears, then do not hesitate to contact your doctor, midwife or health visitor for reassurance and further explanations.

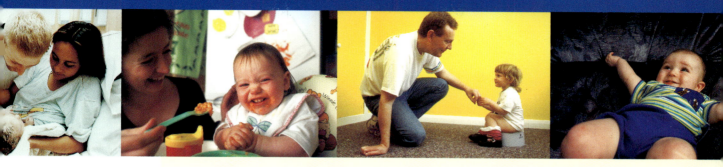

About this book

Welcome to *Ready Steady Baby!* We have produced this book to give clear and up-to-date information about pregnancy, childbirth and caring for your child up to the age of three. We hope that you will enjoy reading it, and will keep it to refer to in the future.

If you want to look up a specific topic, there is an index at the back of the book.

Ready Steady Baby! is written by an experienced author who is also a mother, plus a team of experts. We hope it will answer your questions, and help with any concerns you may have.

Remember that there are many people who will be caring for you and your baby—if you need to talk to anyone in more detail about any aspect of your care, or your baby's health or development, then please don't hesitate to contact your doctor, midwife or health visitor.

Early pregnancy

THE FIRST SIGNS

If you have a regular menstrual cycle, you may notice you miss a period about two weeks after you conceived. You may have other signs as well — you may even be aware of some of them before you notice your missed period, especially if you're hoping to be pregnant, and watching for changes. Arrange a visit to your GP to have your pregnancy confirmed and discuss antenatal care.

Changes within your body occur because of pregnancy hormones, which are released into your bloodstream, and which affect various parts of your body.

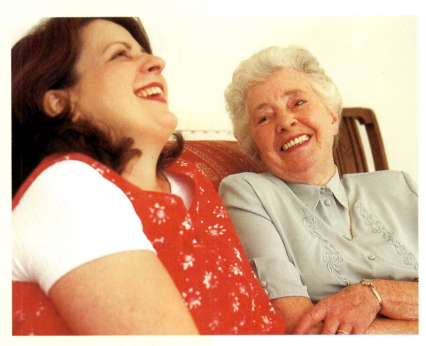

- **Your breasts start to change soon after you conceive.** Your body starts to make tissue for producing and storing milk. You may feel your breasts are more tender than usual. Tiny spots around the nipple area — called tubercles — become more obvious.

- **You may feel sick, and go off certain foods and smells.** Some women do vomit. This usually happens in the mornings, but it can happen at other times as well. A metallic taste in your mouth may affect your sense of taste. The smell of some foods may make you feel unwell.

- **You may feel tired.** Some women say they feel more tired in early pregnancy than at any other time.

- **You may need to pass urine more often.**

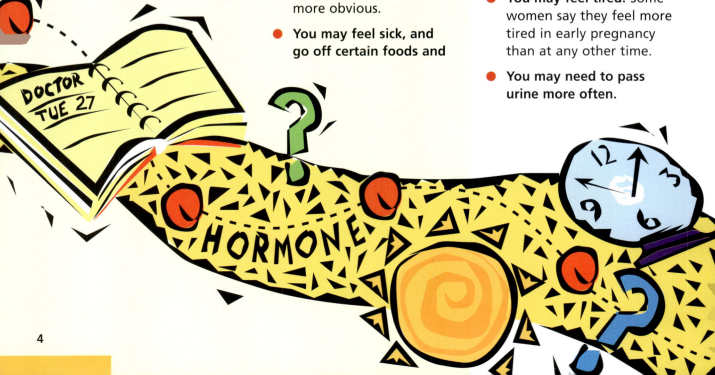

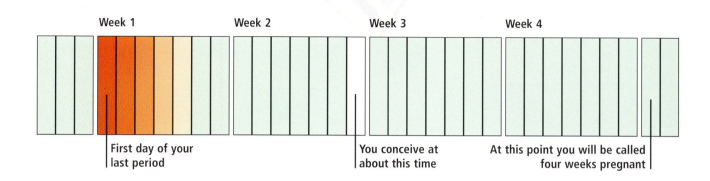

| Week 1 | Week 2 | Week 3 | Week 4 |

First day of your
last period

You conceive at
about this time

At this point you will be called
four weeks pregnant

'I always had an idea I'd be a mum some day, but now it's going to happen, I don't really know what my feelings are. It's come as a shock. I told my boyfriend and he was so pleased. I know he expected me to feel the same. But I can't. I'm hoping I will change — it's early days yet.'

'I'm so excited, I can't wait to tell everyone — I'm looking forward to having a bump so I can look pregnant as well as feel it!'

'I have felt so ill these last three weeks — sick not just in the mornings but in the afternoons and evenings as well — and tired, too. Feeling this bad takes the edge off feeling good about the pregnancy.'

questions answered   Q&A

Q. When is your baby due?

A. Pregnancy usually lasts from 37–42 weeks, or between nine and nine-and-a-half calendar months. This is based on the average length of a menstrual cycle, which is 28 days. The start of your pregnancy is dated from the first day of your last period, even though you conceived after this. If you usually have your period more often, or less often, than every 28 days, the date you expect your baby should take that into account.

- It's helpful to think of the 'due date' as only a rough guide. Very few women (around five per cent) actually give birth on the date they are 'due'. Most babies come at some time during the fortnight before or the fortnight after this date.

- If you don't know when your last period was, your midwife or doctor can use other signs and symptoms to establish the length of your pregnancy. You may also be offered an ultrasound scan.

YOUR IDENTITY AS 'YOU'

Sometimes, you may feel your own identity is lost — the focus is on you as a mother, and not you as a person who has lots of other aspects to her life besides this. But on the whole, the attention you get in pregnancy is warm, and well worth enjoying.

It's usual to have some anxieties about your health or the development of your baby. You'll be thinking ahead to the birth, too. If something is troubling you, you can talk to your midwife about it in confidence. If you don't yet have a telephone number for a midwife, contact your hospital, family doctor or health centre and ask to be put in touch with a midwife.

'People relate to you differently when you're pregnant. I feel my friends are looking forward to the baby, too — everyone's so interested.'

'I feel I've got closer to my mother since becoming pregnant — she's started to share memories of her own pregnancies with me, and we've had some good long chats together.'

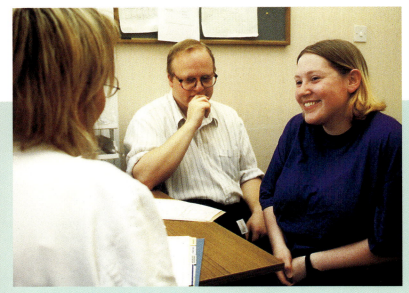

BEING INVOLVED

FATHERS share many of the same feelings as mothers during pregnancy. If you're a father-to-be, you may sometimes be anxious and nervous about your baby's health and your partner's health. You may be delighted, but also wonder what the labour and birth will be like, and how you will cope. Here are some fathers' experiences.

'I found it hard going. Liz was very emotional and touchy in the first few months, partly because we lost a baby two years ago, and she was worried it would happen again. It was quite difficult. Towards the end, things got easier from that aspect, but she had high blood pressure and was told to rest. She needed a lot of support and encouragement.'

'I feel good about being a father — I really do. I love the fact that Yvonne is pregnant, and the way her body is changing. I actually feel proud of her, and of me. There have been times when I have started to think ahead, and I get a bit worried about the changes it will bring, but I think we'll cope. The positives outweigh the negatives.'

6

Fitness & health in pregnancy

What you do, and how you live your life, affects your baby. Making changes can make a difference. A lot of the advice and information in this book will answer many of your questions and help you to care for your health at this important time.

SMOKING

You probably know that smoking can affect your baby now and in the future:

- smoking raises the levels of carbon monoxide in your blood, so that less oxygen will reach your baby

- harmful chemicals reach your baby

- nicotine constricts the blood vessels on your side of the placenta, which means oxygen is passed over less efficiently to the baby.

The result is that the baby grows less well and may be born lighter. Low birth weight may mean problems during and after labour, and the baby may pick up infections more easily. Smoking also affects brain development and the general health of your baby. The effects have been shown to last into childhood, and beyond. There is also evidence that partners who smoke affect the baby's health — whether or not the pregnant woman smokes herself.

If you stop smoking, your baby is:

- less likely to be born before she is ready

- less likely to have breathing problems

- better able to resist infection

- less at risk from cot death, infection and chronic conditions such as asthma.

If you or your partner stop smoking you reduce all of these risks. Toddlers and children grow up healthier in a smoke-free atmosphere.

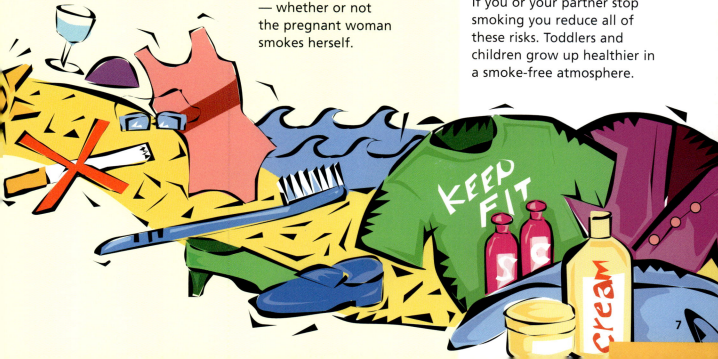

Stop smoking!

Giving up is worthwhile at any time in pregnancy — the sooner the better. Help yourself by:

- giving up with your partner, or a friend

- putting aside the money you have saved, and spending it on a treat

- taking up something you can't do at the same time as smoking — sewing, knitting, or another craft.

It is important to stay stopped once your baby has been born.

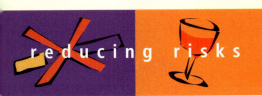

reducing risks

'I stopped just like that. A case of mind over matter. Had two girls and needed cash for other things. They don't smoke and neither do I.'

Ex-smoker with support from Smokeline

ALCOHOL

Some women don't like the taste of alcohol when they're pregnant, so they stop drinking it. If you don't stop, alcohol does reach your baby, but the evidence is that light, occasional drinking — one or two units, once or twice a week — is not likely to do any harm. Heavy drinking is associated with miscarriage, and sometimes with serious effects on your baby's development such as fetal alcohol syndrome.

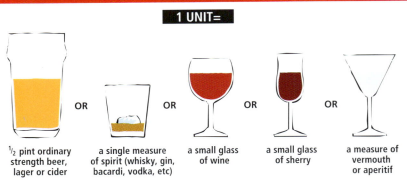

1 UNIT=

¹/₂ pint ordinary strength beer, lager or cider OR a single measure of spirit (whisky, gin, bacardi, vodka, etc) OR a small glass of wine OR a small glass of sherry OR a measure of vermouth or aperitif

These apply to the 25ml measure used in most of England and Wales. In some places, pub measures are larger than this. In Northern Ireland, a pub measure is 35ml — or 1¹/₂ units. In Scotland it can either be 35ml or 25ml. Take care—home measures are usually larger than these standard ones!

DRUGS

Any drugs may affect you or your growing baby — including illegal or street drugs. Always tell your doctor you are pregnant if you are prescribed any medication. If you buy medicines at the chemist's, ask the pharmacist if it's okay to take the product in pregnancy. Check the label yourself, as well.

- Cocaine, crack, heroin, amphetamines and cannabis are known to affect a baby directly and indirectly. Crack and cocaine are especially dangerous, as they have an immediate effect on the baby's blood supply.

Babies of drug-dependent mothers are born dependent themselves, and suffer from withdrawal symptoms at birth.

- If you cannot stop using any drug, seek help. Some maternity units have specialist addiction units. Being pregnant may be the extra encouragement you need to cope with giving up. Your midwife, health visitor or antenatal clinic can put you in touch with support services, or speak to your family doctor.

See also **Further help** at the back of this book (page 151).

Q. How can I avoid everything that might harm my baby? Exhaust fumes, pollution, radiation — they're everywhere. Is it possible to be completely safe?

A. You can't avoid everything that's harmful, but it makes sense to do what you can. The risk to your baby from smoking, for instance, is not just a theory. The effects have been demonstrated by good research. Worrying about aspects of your life which you can't control or avoid isn't very productive. It's worth remembering that the vast majority of babies are born strong and healthy.

Q. What about herbal medicine or homoeopathic remedies? And is aromatherapy safe?

A. Most homoeopathic remedies are generally considered to be very safe in pregnancy, but check with the prescriber or pharmacist. Some herbal medicines and some aromatherapy oils are not suitable for pregnant women. If you prefer to take these products, get advice from a properly qualified practitioner. For minor complaints, there are useful books which will tell you what to avoid in pregnancy.

'Both of us have been smokers for about ten years, and I've never managed to give up for more than a few weeks before. This time, though, I think I will stay off. Joe has stopped smoking in the house, and I hope he'll soon stop completely... it's hard, but it's got to be worth trying.'

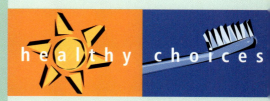

healthy choices

Your partner can help you and your baby stay healthy by stopping smoking. If this isn't possible straight away, make a start by smoking away from the house only.

For more advice on smoking, alcohol or drugs see your midwife, GP or health visitor. If you want to stop smoking contact:

smokeline on 0800 84 84 84

for free information and support for you and for your partner.

Avoid X-rays in pregnancy if possible. This includes dental X-rays.

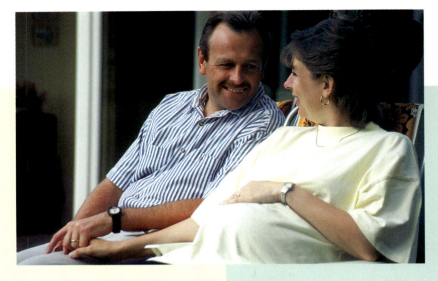

YOUR BODY IS CHANGING

Sometimes you may feel tired, run down and uncomfortable. At other times, though, you'll feel you really know what people mean when they talk about the 'bloom' of pregnancy.

- Pregnancy hormones can change your skin and hair. Oily skin can become oilier, and dry skin can become drier, so skin care routines and hair care may change.

- From the fourth or fifth month, hormones affect the colour of your skin. The darker your skin, the more you'll notice it. If you have very fair skin and red hair, you may not. Nipples get darker, and the areola (the area around the nipple) gets bigger. A linea nigra ('black line') may appear down the midline of your chest and abdomen. Patchy colour may appear on your face. Using sunbeds is not advisable at any time but in pregnancy this patchy effect could be made worse by the sunbed. Be careful to use protection on your skin when outside in the sun.

- Stretchmarks are reddish-coloured stripes on the abdomen, breasts and thighs. They appear when the underlying tissues of the skin are stretched. After pregnancy, they gradually fade to a silvery-grey. The skin's elasticity is, to a large extent, inherited. Creams and lotions won't make much difference, although they are pleasant to use. Their moisturising effect keeps the surface of your skin free from itching and dryness.

Take care of your feet. You may be most comfortable in low-heeled or flat shoes. High heels can make any backache you have worse. Your feet may swell because your body retains more fluid, so you may need a wider fitting shoe, or even a half size larger. You may also have puffy ankles, and some aching. Some fluid retention is normal in pregnancy, but you should tell your midwife or doctor if there is any sudden increase.

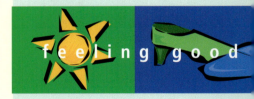

National Health Service (NHS) dental treatment, prescriptions and chiropody are free while you are pregnant (and for a year after the birth). However, you need a certificate, issued by your health board. Ask your midwife or family doctor.

EXERCISE IN PREGNANCY

Exercising to keep active and fit helps you feel well, so that you're in good physical condition for the birth. Exercise improves your heart's functioning and your circulation, which will help common complaints of pregnancy such as constipation, varicose veins or swelling (oedema). If you have backache, exercise and some attention to your posture can do a lot to relieve it.

Walking, swimming, some forms of yoga, or tone and stretch, can be done at any stage of pregnancy. It's best to avoid sports or exercise with a risk of falling, or hard physical contact with other players. Any exercises which 'bounce' your baby on your pelvic floor may also cause long-term damage to these muscles.

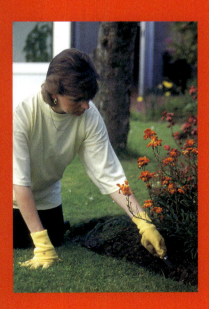

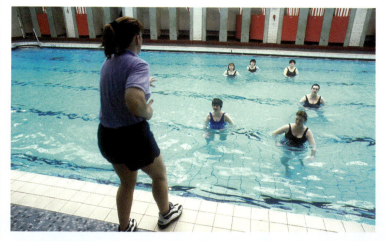

Swimming

Even if you haven't done much exercise before your pregnancy, you'll find swimming is easy. The water supports your whole body, so there's almost no risk of injury, and you can tone and stretch all over.

● Many pools run 'aquanatal' classes, where you learn movements and exercises designed for pregnancy. These should be run by a specially trained midwife, or an obstetric physiotherapist with a midwife present.

● In any class, you should be given the chance to warm up with some gentle limb stretches, followed by movements which work round the body, and maybe a swim.

questions Q&A answered

Q. I do aerobics twice or three times a week. Is it safe now I'm pregnant?

A. If you're already used to aerobics, then carry on. Tell your instructor you are pregnant, and avoid doing any exercises which risk straining your back. After about five months, concentrate on stretching and toning, without any jogging or jumping.

Remember to watch out for any exercises that might 'bounce' your baby onto your pelvic floor. Don't do any abdominal sit-up exercises. Stop before you feel really tired. This isn't the time for anyone to start doing this form of exercise.

Yoga

Yoga is generally a safe and helpful form of exercise in pregnancy. The poses gently stretch the body, and the breathing methods and emphasis on relaxation encourage peace and calm.

- If you belong to a class, tell the teacher you are pregnant. If you want to start yoga, it's best to find a teacher rather than try by yourself. Local authority adult education classes usually include yoga courses.

- Some of the very advanced poses will be beyond you in pregnancy, and you shouldn't attempt them. Just as with any exercise, stop if you feel any strain.

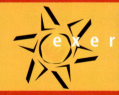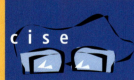

Loosen up!

Your pelvis needs to 'open up' to allow the baby to get through during labour and birth. To allow this, the ligaments in your pelvis soften and become more stretchable. Hormones, including relaxin, help this to happen.

Ligaments are bands of strong, elastic-like tissue connecting the bones of your skeleton at the joints. Because your ligaments soften in pregnancy, it's easy to stretch too far and end up straining a ligament — especially if you're not used to exercise. If you over-stretch you feel pain. This is your body telling you to stop.

Stand tall!

You can strengthen your back, and avoid backache, by learning to 'stand tall'. Stand with feet apart and let the weight of the body sink through to your feet. Imagine a string from the top of your head drawing you up towards the ceiling. Feel your spine lengthening.

- If you have to stand, remember this posture. It helps to stop you slumping and sagging into your tummy.

- Try not to sit for long periods of time. When sitting, tuck a small cushion into the small of your back to help you sit straight and comfortably. This takes the strain away from your back.

Eating in pregnancy

FOODS TO CHOOSE, FOODS TO AVOID

Healthy eating in pregnancy is no different from healthy eating at any other time of your life. If you already eat well, you don't have to make any major changes in pregnancy. There are only a few, potentially important, points to watch in the foods you choose, and in the way you prepare your food before eating it. (See page 16 for further information on vegetarian and vegan diets.)

Foods to choose

Healthy eating doesn't mean you have to eat anything you don't enjoy. Aim to eat foods from each of these food groups:

- **bread, cereals, rice, pasta, potatoes** — these should make up the main part of every meal. Wholegrain cereal foods such as brown rice or wholemeal bread have more fibre and are more filling.

- **fruit and vegetables** — try to aim for five or more portions of fruit and vegetables per day. Use any kind, including fresh, frozen, tinned and dried, and pure fruit juices.

- **meat, fish and alternatives (these provide protein and iron)** — include some food from this group twice a day. This includes meat, chicken, fish (including tinned fish), eggs, nuts (see important note over the page), beans, pulses.

- **milk and dairy foods (these provide an important source of calcium)** — try to include one pint of milk per day or swap $1/3$ of a pint of milk for 1oz of cheese (matchbox size), a yoghurt or a bowl of milk pudding. Low fat dairy products have the same amount of calcium as full fat varieties.

- **foods containing fat and foods containing sugar** — keep foods from this group to a minimum.

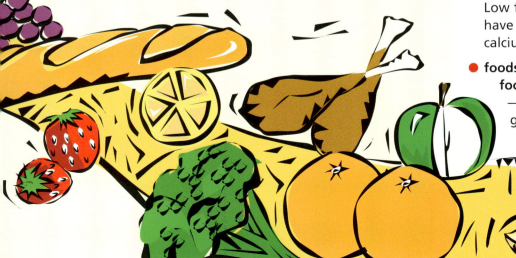

13

Foods to avoid

Some foods do carry risks in pregnancy. The risks are very small, so even if you do eat some of these foods, perhaps without realising, you are unlikely to harm yourself or your baby in any way. But it makes sense to avoid them if you can. Certain foods may be contaminated with bacteria such as listeria and salmonella.

Foods to avoid are:

- unpasteurised milks
- soft, ripened cheeses (such as brie, camembert and similar blue-veined varieties)
- liver and liver products (see page 15)
- pâtés — all types
- raw and undercooked eggs (cook until both the white and yolk are solid)
- ice-cream from soft whip machines (**Note**: wrapped or block ice-cream is safe)
- mayonnaise (homemade)
- shark, marlin and swordfish. Tuna should be restricted to two medium cans or one fresh steak per week. This follows concerns about mercury in these fish and also applies to women who are breastfeeding or intending to become pregnant.

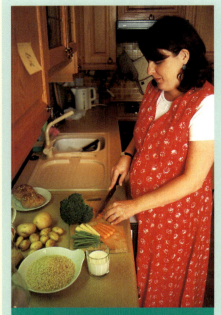

GENERAL HYGIENE

- Always wash your hands before and after handling any food.

- Wash all fruit and vegetables, including ready-prepared salads, thoroughly before eating.

- Wash your hands after handling raw meat.

- Store raw foods separately from prepared foods.

- Always wear gloves and wash your hands thoroughly after gardening or handling soil.

CONTACT WITH ANIMALS

Some animals, particularly cats and sheep, may carry harmful micro-organisms including listeria, chlamydia psittaci or toxoplasma. These organisms can cause infection in pregnant women and cause harm to the unborn child.

- Always wash your hands after stroking your pet, especially before eating and preparing food.

- Try to keep pets out of the kitchen, and particularly off any surface on which you prepare food.

- Use separate dishes and utensils for preparing pet food and clean them separately from your family's.

- Keep your cat litter tray clean. Try to get someone else to dispose of soiled litter. If you have to handle it always wear rubber gloves **and** wash your hands and the gloves thoroughly afterwards.

- Always wear gloves when gardening in case cats have fouled in the garden. Wash your hands thoroughly afterwards.

Source: *While You Are Pregnant*, pp. 7–8, Department of Health, 1995.

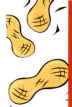

If you or members of your close family suffer from peanut allergy or allergic disease such as atopic eczema, asthma or hayfever, it is recommended that you should avoid eating peanuts or foods containing peanut products during pregnancy and whilst breastfeeding.

FOLIC ACID

Folic acid is one of the important B vitamins. It's found naturally in many foods, and is added to some manufactured foods. This vitamin is vital for the growth and health of all the cells in the body. Folic acid is very important in the early stages of pregnancy, or if you are planning a pregnancy.

Women planning a pregnancy and pregnant women should take more folic acid to help prevent babies from being affected by 'neural tube defects' such as spina bifida.

Currently, it's recommended you take a 400 mcg (0.4 mg) folic acid tablet for at least three months before becoming pregnant and for 12 weeks into your pregnancy.

If you become pregnant unexpectedly, start taking a folic acid tablet every day until the twelfth week.

How to take it

If you are planning to become pregnant, or as soon as you know you are pregnant:

- start taking a daily supplement in the form of a 400 mcg folic acid tablet (the recommended dose), which your doctor may prescribe, or which you can buy in pharmacies and some supermarkets

  and

- eat more foods that contain folic acid.

> Avoid taking Vitamin A supplements as high levels could be harmful to the baby. Your doctor will prescribe vitamin supplements if you need them.

Foods with folic acid

- Green vegetables, including spinach, broccoli, green beans, cauliflower, Brussels sprouts, peas.

- Cereal foods, including bread. Some breads and breakfast cereals are fortified with folic acid — check the label.

- Some fruits, including oranges, grapefruit, bananas.

- Beans and pulses, especially black-eyed beans, chick peas.

- Milk and yoghurt.

- Yeast extracts (taken as a drink or a spread).

> ## What about liver?
> Liver contains folic acid but also has high levels of Vitamin A, which could be harmful to the baby in the early months of pregnancy. Pregnant women, and women planning a pregnancy, are advised not to eat liver, or liver products.

DIFFERENT TASTES?

Changes in how you feel about certain foods during your pregnancy is common. You may find you cannot take some foods and drinks which you previously enjoyed, like coffee or alcohol. Similarly you may find you have an increased liking for other foods, some of which you may not have enjoyed before becoming pregnant, eg citrus fruits and milk. Some women develop a taste for odd combinations of food. As long as you are eating a healthy balance of foods (see page 13), increasing the amount you eat of one food or cutting out another will not matter. If your craving is for very sweet or high fat foods, like chocolate, try to keep the amount you eat in moderation.

Q. I was overweight before becoming pregnant. Is it okay to try to slim while I am pregnant?

A. Don't aim to lose weight when you're pregnant. Instead, aim for a healthy balance of foods. Discuss this with your midwife or GP. Remember foods containing fat and foods containing sugar can provide a lot of calories (energy) and should be kept to a minimum.

Q. Is a vegetarian or vegan diet safe in pregnancy?

A. Yes, as long as you follow all the guidelines for healthy eating. All the nutrients you need are available in foods other than meat. Vegans — who eat no food from animal sources — may need extra Vitamin B12, and should choose foods such as soya products which have been fortified with Vitamin B12, or take supplements.

See also **Further help** at the back of this book.

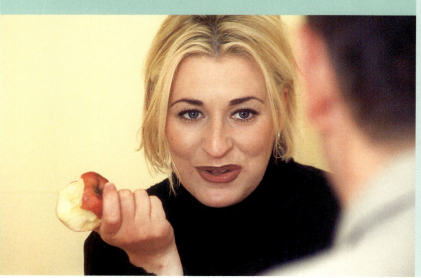

Weeks up to 6

CONCEPTION AND EARLY PREGNANCY

This is the most 'active' part of your baby's development. A great deal happens in these first weeks — often before you know for sure you are pregnant.

- **The fertilised egg — now called a blastocyst — attaches itself to the womb lining** by the end of the first week after fertilisation. It burrows into the lining, and there is an exchange of chemicals and nutrients between the blastocyst and the lining.

- **When the blastocyst is well-implanted it is known as the embryo** and is about the same size as the full stop at the end of this sentence.

- **The outer cells of the embryo start to attach themselves to the mother's blood vessels,**

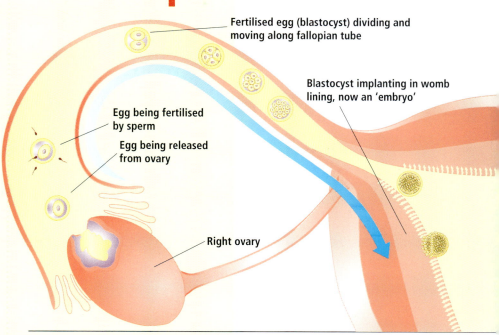

Fertilised egg (blastocyst) dividing and moving along fallopian tube

Egg being fertilised by sperm

Egg being released from ovary

Blastocyst implanting in womb lining, now an 'embryo'

Right ovary

linking in to the mother's blood supply. This is the beginning of the chorionic villi, which will become the placenta.

- **The inner cells of the embryo then divide into three separate layers.** The first layer will become the nervous system and brain; the second layer will become major internal organs (digestive system and lungs); the third layer will become the heart and the blood system, the muscles and the skeleton.

- **The embryo now has its own blood vessels.** Some of them connect with your own blood supply in the uterine wall. They develop into the umbilical cord, which contains the blood vessels taking nutrients from the placenta, and waste products from the baby.

When you are six weeks pregnant, this very complex organism is about the same size as the nail on your little finger.

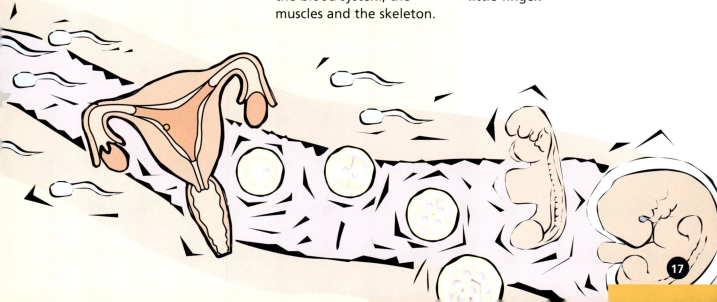

WEEKS 4–5

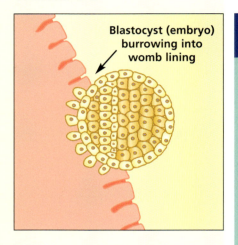

Blastocyst (embryo) burrowing into womb lining

You may have slight bleeding around the time when the egg implants itself into the wall of the uterus. It's easy to mistake this for a very light period, so you may not realise you are pregnant.

WEEK 6

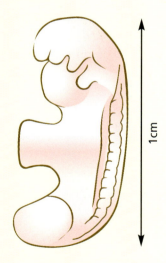

1cm

The baby's heartbeat can be detected on a scan as early as six or seven weeks.

questions Q&A answered

Q. Are pregnancy tests really all that reliable? I was sure I was pregnant, but the test showed negative. A week later I did it again and it was positive.

A. Pregnancy tests are usually reliable when used properly, though there is a small chance of a false negative. The tests you buy at the chemist's can pick up the hormone human chorionic gonadotrophin (HCG) in urine from about two weeks after conception ie at about the time when you would be due a period. But sometimes there may not be quite enough HCG present for the test to detect, which is why you should repeat the test if your period still doesn't come. This hormone can also be detected in a blood test.

OTHER SIGNS OF PREGNANCY

- Your cervix softens slightly.
- The vagina and the cervix change colour — from pink to purplish-blue — because of the increased blood supply in these areas.
- Your breasts start to change, and the tubercles (small, spot-like bumps) on the areola (area surrounding the nipple) become more prominent. These tubercles are the exit points of glands which produce an oily substance to keep the nipples supple and soft, in preparation for breastfeeding.

Take folic acid supplements for at least the first 12 weeks of pregnancy (see page 15).

Weeks 7–12

TAKING SHAPE

Now the embryo starts to develop a human body shape, and the major organs develop.

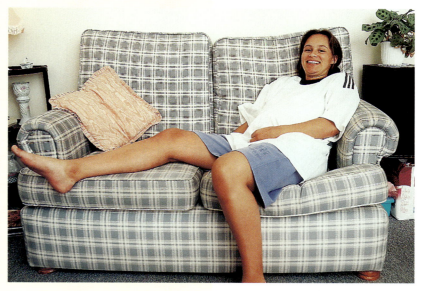

- Within a couple of weeks, there are small bumps called **limb buds**, which become arms and legs.

- By week 10, there is a larger, rounded end which will become the head. The umbilical cord has lengthened, and the embryo is floating inside the **amniotic sac** (the 'bag of waters' which protects the baby throughout the pregnancy).

- At the end of this time, the embryo is called a **fetus**. Facial features start to form — mouth, tongue and eyelids. The limb buds are now recognisable arms and legs, with the beginnings of the fingers and toes. Important work in forming the internal organs, the brain and the nervous system and the skeleton happens in these weeks. By the end of 12 weeks, the structure of the internal organs is complete, and the muscles begin to develop. At the end of week 12, the baby measures about 5 cm (1.9 inches) from head to bottom — the size of a ripe plum.

- By 12 weeks you may find your waistline is already thickening. The organs in the pelvis are being slightly displaced as your uterus moves upwards. You may have some fluid retention, too, which makes you feel fuller around your middle. You won't look pregnant to most people, though.

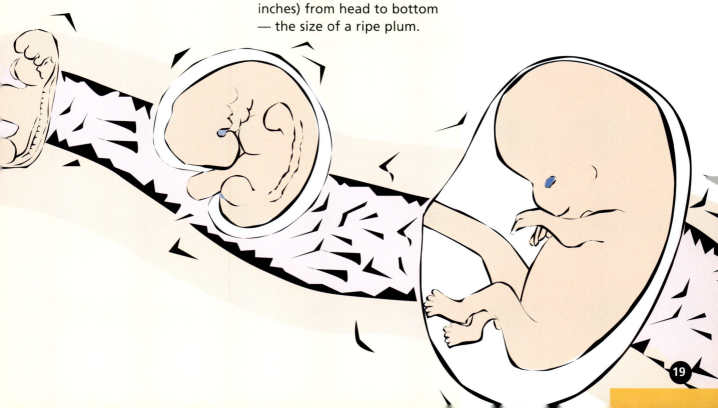

SICKNESS AND NAUSEA

In the first 12 weeks, sickness and nausea may be at its worst. You may feel very tired, too. You are likely to feel better soon. Hormones change at about 12 to 14 weeks, when the placenta starts working, and most women feel better after this.

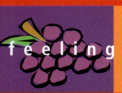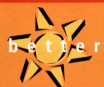

feeling better

What to do

- Keep meals small and frequent, so your stomach always has something in it.

- Start the day with a dry cracker and a drink — even before you get out of bed.

- Avoid the foods and smells that make you feel unwell.

- Ask your GP or your midwife for more suggestions.

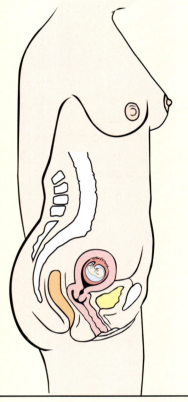

WEEK 9

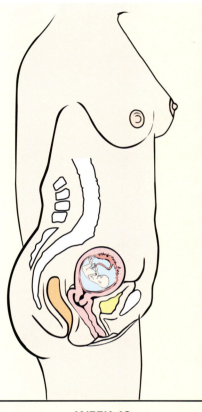

WEEK 12

The fetus is becoming more human in appearance.

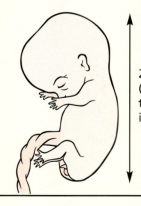

2 cm (less than an inch)

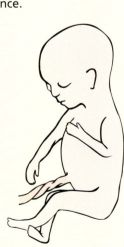

Weeks 13–16

The placenta starts to take over as the main source of nourishment for the baby from week 13. It functions fully by week 14.

YOUR BABY'S FEATURES

- At the beginning of these weeks, the baby has some independent movement of the limbs and the head, though you won't feel it yet. You might feel some movement at 16 weeks, often later in first pregnancies.

- By week 16, your baby's face has clearly marked eyes, nose, mouth and ears. The eyelids have developed, and the teeth are inside the gums.

- There is a soft, fine covering of hair all over the body, called 'lanugo'.

- If your baby is going to have dark hair, the cells of the hair follicles which produce colour begin to work from week 15.

- Eyebrows and eyelashes also start to grow. Fingernails and toenails are there. The eyes and ears continue to develop, and we know babies at this stage are aware of sound and light.

At week 16, your baby is 8 cm (about 3 inches) in length.

THE PLACENTA

This is your baby's life-support system. It is attached to the uterus on one side, and to the baby by the umbilical cord on the other. The umbilical cord brings nutrients from the mother's blood via the placenta to the baby and carries waste products away. The placenta also produces hormones which circulate around your body.

Your bloodstream and your baby's never normally come into direct contact. Your blood bathes the side of the placenta attached to the uterus wall. Nutrients, including oxygen, pass through a membrane which separates your bloodstream from the baby's, then into the baby's bloodstream on the other side of the placenta. Waste products from the baby are dealt with in the same way, passing from the baby's side to your side through the membrane.

The placenta filters out many hazards before they can reach the baby. However, some harmful substances can

still get through the barrier. The placenta can't 'block' some bacteria, viruses, some drugs and medicines, nicotine and carbon monoxide.

The hormones produced by the placenta — mainly oestrogen and progesterone — bring about many of the changes you can observe in your body during pregnancy.

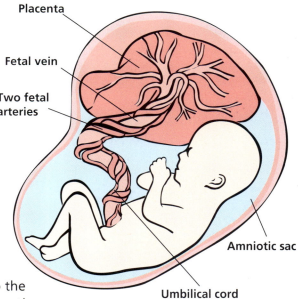

Placenta

Fetal vein

Two fetal arteries

Amniotic sac

Umbilical cord

They affect the growth of your uterus and cause new blood vessels to develop. At the end of pregnancy, the levels of progesterone produced by the placenta fall, but it is not entirely clear what is responsible for starting labour.

Weeks 17–20

YOUR 'BUMP' SHOWS

During these weeks, you start to look pregnant, although women who are very slim and who have a small 'bump' may not look very different, especially if they wear loose clothing.

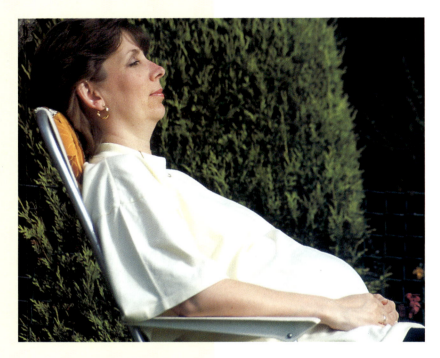

- Around now, you will probably feel the baby's first movements — though you may not be sure that's what they are, especially if you have never been pregnant before. The movements (known as 'quickening') feel fluttery at first, but as time goes on you will feel them as definite pokes and prods, as your baby's movements touch the inside of your abdomen.

- Ultrasound pictures have shown babies of about 18 weeks sucking their thumbs.

- Your baby's second teeth begin to form, behind the start of the first teeth. The baby's body begins to be covered in 'vernix', a greasy substance which coats your baby's skin forming a waterproof layer.

- At 20 weeks, your baby is 15 cm in length (about 6 inches), still small enough to curl into an adult hand.

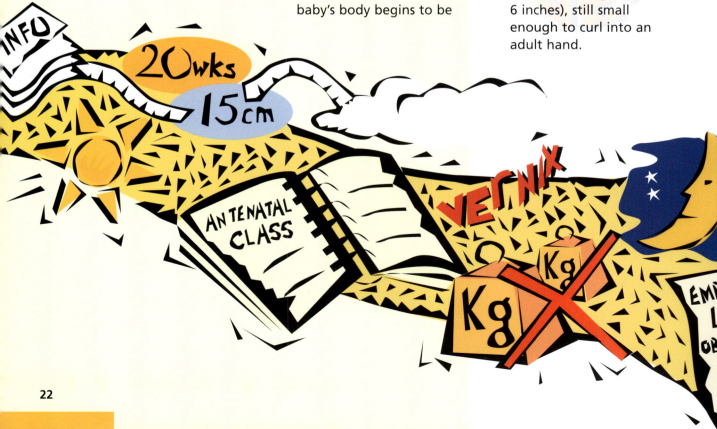

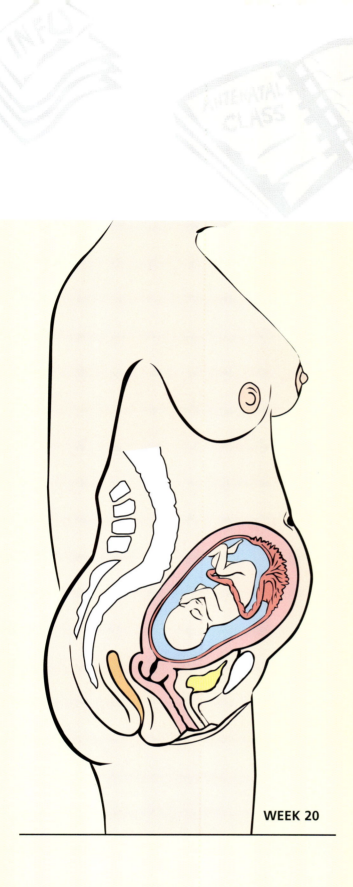

WEEK 20

WORKING DURING PREGNANCY

Most pregnant women are able to work as long as they want to. However, a very few jobs may be unsafe or ill-advised when you're pregnant.

● If you work with **chemicals**, for example, or other dangerous substances, or if your job involves **climbing, or lifting heavy weights**, you may have to switch the tasks you do for something safer. Ask your midwife or doctor for their advice.

● **Your employer has a legal obligation** to make sure the work you do, and your working conditions, will not put your health, or your baby's, at risk. If there is a risk, he or she must offer you alternative employment.

● **You are entitled to paid time off** to attend antenatal appointments and antenatal classes. (You may have to produce a note from your doctor or midwife stating that these classes are considered to be part of your antenatal care.)

● **Start thinking about benefits**, if you haven't already, and about whether or not you intend to go back to work after your baby's born. You can find sources of information about money matters and your maternity rights in the **Further help** section at the back of this book. (See also page 57.)

Weeks 21–24

CHANGING SHAPE

At this time, your uterus grows rapidly and you may gain quite a bit of weight. At about 24 weeks, you'll notice your tummy button flattening, or even popping out, with the pressure from the growing uterus beneath.

MEASURING THE BABY

During antenatal appointments, the midwife or doctor may measure your tummy with a tape. They will also feel (palpate) your tummy with their hands to check the baby's size and growth. The position will be noted. Babies change their position all the time, right up to a few weeks before the birth.

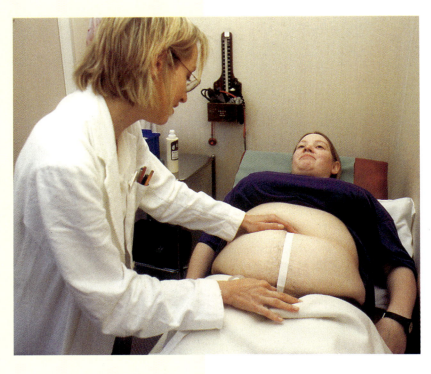

FEELING BETTER

Many women begin to feel energetic and fit, as the tiredness common in early pregnancy goes, and you don't yet feel the heaviness of late pregnancy. Although you may feel tired, you'll probably sleep well and wake refreshed. Your body is doing a lot of unseen work — for example, your heart and lungs are actually working 50 per cent harder than when you're not pregnant.

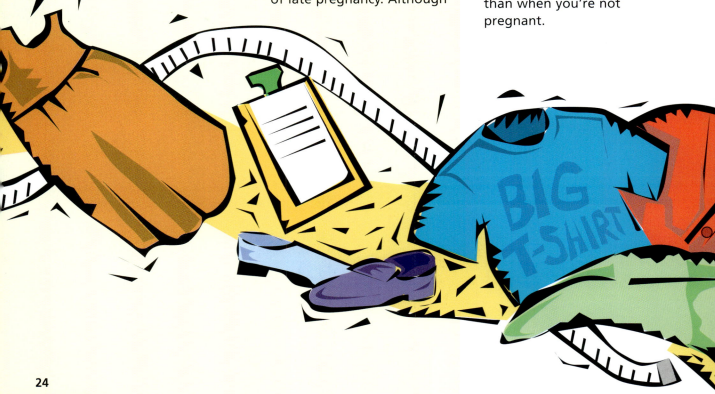

BIG T-SHIRT

MATERNITY CLOTHES — DO YOU NEED THEM?

After about four or five months, you won't fit into many of your ordinary clothes, as your waist thickens, and your breasts get larger. If you buy clothes, try to choose things you can wear afterwards — roomy, loose tops, sweaters and T-shirts. You may find you need to buy one or two special items in the very last weeks, if you get very big. Here are some more ideas pregnant

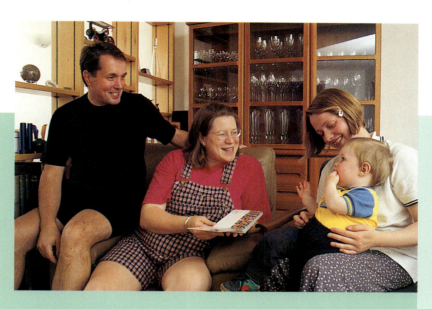

women have suggested to help:

- **maternity leggings** are a good buy — you can wear them after the birth, too, replacing the elastic in the waistband if necessary with a shorter length

- **large T-shirts, shirts and jumpers**. Men's sizes are roomy and comfortable if you don't mind rolling up extra long sleeves

- **wear ordinary tights** (cheaper than maternity ones) but buy them in extra large sizes and wear them back to front, so the larger part of the pants is over your tummy

- **most women feel more comfortable in a bra**, even if they don't normally wear one. Get measured for a maternity bra at about seven months. Nursing bras have cups which unhook or unzip, and are helpful for breastfeeding later.

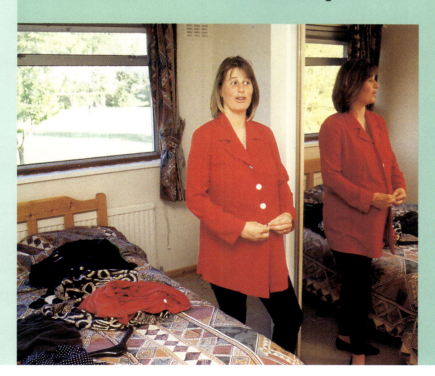

Weeks 25–28

YOUR DEVELOPING BABY

Your baby's body gradually looks more in proportion and baby-like during these weeks.

- You'll feel your baby move a lot more, and you may see movements if you lie still in the bath. You might even be able to make out which movements come from a hand or a foot, especially later on, when the uterus is larger.

- The skin is less transparent now and starts to thicken. Babies of this age have hardly any fat under their skin, so it is wrinkled and loose. Creases appear on the palms of the hands and the soles of feet, and by the end of 25 weeks fingerprints form.

- Although not common, babies are sometimes born this early. Today, with specialist care, babies can survive outside the uterus from as early as 24 weeks of pregnancy. Great progress has been made in this area of medicine in the last few years. However, at this early stage many babies who survive can have long-term problems.

Survival rates increase week-by-week after this time. Most babies born at 28 weeks survive without long-term problems, though they still need weeks of special care.

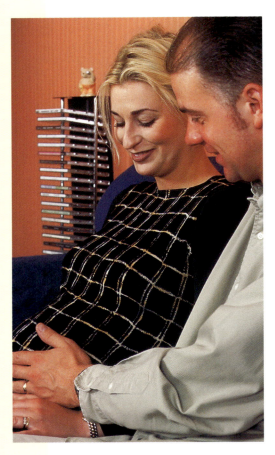

- At 28 weeks, your baby is about 22 cm long (8½ inches), and weighs 800 grams (about one-and-a-half pounds).

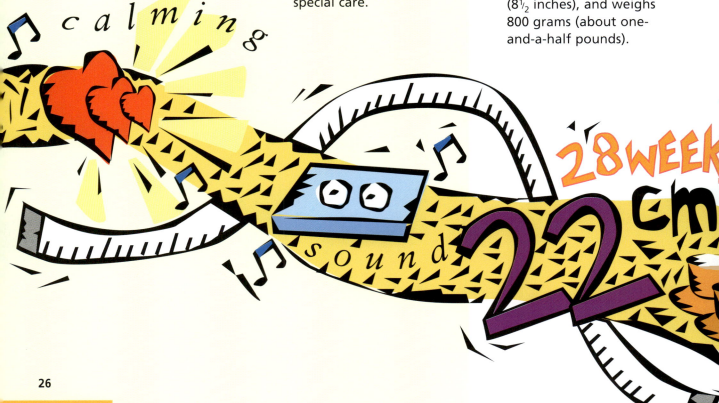

CHANGES

- Your breasts produce **colostrum** (a thick, creamy substance) at this time, though you may not be aware of it. This is the first fluid made in your breasts (see page 92). Some women leak a little. If you notice this, it's nothing to worry about. It will dry into small crusts on your nipples, so just wash this off with plain water.

- There may be some **oedema** (swelling) of your feet and hands. This is very common from 26 weeks or so onwards. You should point it out next time you see your midwife or doctor. It's not likely to be anything more serious than the normal fluid retention of pregnancy (see page 53). But severe oedema plus high blood pressure and protein in the urine would suggest you have pre-eclampsia (see pages 55–56) and this is more important.

questions Q&A answered

Q. I get very stressed at work, and sometimes at home, too. I then feel guilty in case my baby picks it up.

A. If you are feeling very stressed or tired, then do take steps to reduce it. You might benefit from resting more, or leaving work early. Or begin your maternity leave sooner than you planned. Recent research shows that high stress levels in pregnancy may affect some aspects of your baby's development, and may also be linked with breathing problems at birth.

YOUR BABY CAN HEAR

Your baby's ears are very sensitive from the 24th week of pregnancy. Inside the uterus, your heartbeat, the noises of your digestive system, your voice and other voices are all heard by your baby. It's well-known that the regular sound of something like a heartbeat can calm a crying newborn. A baby who cries a lot may find womb noises soothing (you can buy a tape).

Weeks 29–32

TIRED AND UNCOMFORTABLE?

From week 30 or so, your baby's body gradually fills out as fat develops underneath the skin. By 30 weeks, the hair on the face and body will start to disappear, but the 'vernix' (see page 22) remains.

Baby boys' testes may descend from their abdomen towards the top of the scrotum from about week 29.

- Now you may start to feel the pressure on your stomach and under your ribs, and on your bladder. This means it can be harder to get into a position where you can breathe easily while lying or sitting, and it means you may need to pass urine more often.

- The skin on your abdomen will feel thin and stretched. This is the time when you might see your first stretchmarks, if you're going to get them (see page 10).

- Stay at work if you want to, as long as your job, or travelling to and from it, is not too physically demanding. Check with your midwife if you're not sure about this. You might prefer to be at home, preparing for your baby

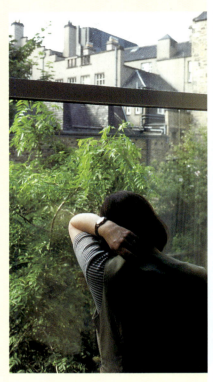

and enjoying the free time you have left if this is your first baby. It may be the longest time to yourself you'll have for quite some time!

- Backache may be more of a problem at this time, as the increasing size of your abdomen draws you forward.

- Your antenatal checks are likely to continue fortnightly at about this time. Some women have an ultrasound scan at some time during these weeks, mainly to see the growth and development of your baby, and to see if the major organs are as they should be.

SEX IN PREGNANCY

Sex is normally perfectly safe in pregnancy. Any sexual activity that doesn't harm you will not harm your baby. You don't risk 'jostling', hurting or affecting your baby. The baby is protected in the uterus by the bag of waters, which cushions movement. The baby may feel the movements of vigorous sexual activity, but they won't do any harm.

Is it ever risky?

Occasionally, women who have had a number of miscarriages might be advised not to have sex around about the time their period would have been due, or even at all during the first three months. There's no evidence that sex and miscarriage are linked, though, and there is some disagreement among doctors about how to advise couples in this situation.

- Some women feel that sex with man or woman on top positions is a little uncomfortable in later pregnancy. You can get round this by the person on top bearing their weight on their arms. Or, try side-by-side positions.

- Some women — and some men — get less keen on penetrative sex as the pregnancy develops. That's fine. You can have closeness and as much sexual excitement as you want without it.

- Women, like men, sometimes find their desire for sex changes in pregnancy, and both men and women may go off it, too.

None of this can mean anything serious, or long-lasting. Try to keep your closeness with lots of warm, physical contact that need not lead to sex. If it played an important role in your lives before, then the feelings are very likely to come back in time.

Your antenatal care appointments have probably been about every four weeks, but they may become fortnightly now, and you may have stopped work. Many antenatal or parentcraft classes start about now (see pages 64–65).

BABIES BORN EARLY: YOUR BABY IN SPECIAL CARE

Babies born before 37 weeks are called 'pre-term' (more usual these days than 'premature'). They usually need some time in the hospital's special or intensive care baby unit. Intensive care is for sicker or weaker babies, who need more medical and nursing support.

- The outlook for pre-term babies is better than it used to be, but being born too soon does bring problems. The main hazards are infection and difficulties with breathing.

- It can be hard to feel your baby is really yours while in an incubator, attached to electrodes and tubes. If your baby is very sick, or very pre-term, you may even be wary of getting too close emotionally, fearing, perhaps, that your baby may not survive.

- You can do a great deal for your baby, though. Even the tiniest pre-term babies can sometimes be cuddled for short times outside the incubator. Touching, stroking, talking to your baby, whether inside or outside the incubator, is important. Studies show that babies who have this sort of loving contact put on weight more quickly. As soon as you can, hold your baby close, with plenty of skin-to-skin contact.

- Staff can explain the machines involved in your baby's care. Some of the equipment simply measures responses and functions, such as breathing, body temperature and heart rate.

- Some babies may be too small or weak to feed from the breast. Even if you didn't intend to breastfeed, you may be asked to express milk for your pre-term baby, to be given through a feeding tube or a little cup. If you plan to carry on breastfeeding, expressing milk will help to establish a milk supply by stimulating your breasts. You can hand express or use an electric pump (see page 98).

- You may not get very much milk at first, but tiny babies only need very small amounts. Your milk is very valuable (see page 93), as the **antibodies** in it help your baby fight infection. The colostrum which the breasts produce in the first days is especially nutritious.

For further information turn to page 67.

Weeks 33–36

GETTING READY

Your baby puts on about 200 grams a week (about seven ounces) in these weeks, growing bigger and laying down more fat.

- After about 33 weeks, you may sometimes feel jerky movements. This is thought to be the baby having a mild attack of hiccups.

- By 36 weeks, most babies (about 95 per cent) are head-down in the uterus, in the position known as 'cephalic'. First babies engage in the pelvis at about this time. The head descends into the pelvis, fitting in quite firmly. Second or later babies tend to engage later (this is because the pelvic bones are arranged slightly differently after a pregnancy and birth). For more information about engagement, see page 32.

- At 36 weeks, your baby measures about 44 cm (18 inches) and weighs 2500 grams (about five-and-a-half pounds).

Packing your bag: some ideas

A few weeks before your expected day of delivery, check that you have the right things to take with you into hospital. It might help to have three bags — one for labour, one for after the birth and one for going home. Your midwife or antenatal clinic may give you a suggestions sheet. If not, here are some.

Preparing for a home birth

If you are planning a home birth your midwife will have a special delivery pack which she will drop off at your house some time before your baby is due. It contains things like sterile cloths and swabs. She will bring her own equipment to the birth. Ask her what she wants you to provide.

Bag one (labour)

- Drinks and snacks for you and your partner.
- Mineral water spray or a plant spray with a fine nozzle. Put it in a fridge (if you have access to one) to keep it cool.
- Two facecloths for cooling your face and skin.
- Music tapes and a cassette player (battery operated).
- Oil or a light body lotion for massage.
- Thermal pack (the sort you can heat in a microwave for taking with you on cold outings or on a picnic — it stays warm for hours). It can be wrapped in a towel and used as a warm compress to relieve aches in the back or in the legs.
- Old nightdress (front-opening for easy breastfeeding) or old T-shirt.
- Dressing-gown (robe) and sandals or slippers.
- Pair of socks.
- Hair brush.
- Hair bands for long hair.
- Wash bag with toiletries and flannel.
- Phone card/coins.

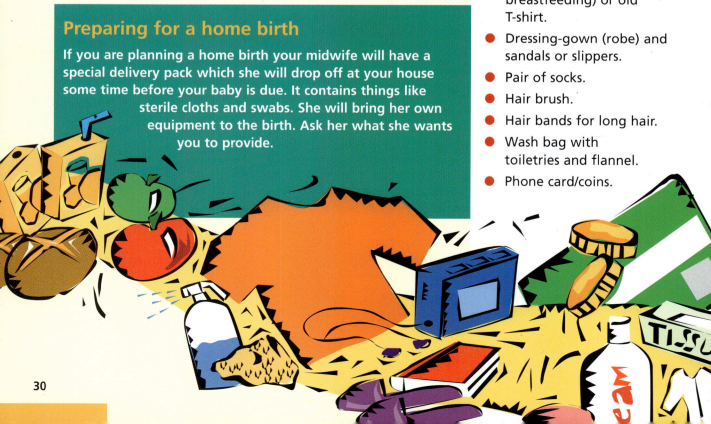

Bag two
(after the birth)

- Two nightdresses (front-opening for easy breastfeeding).
- Easy-to-wear dayclothes (like a jogging suit).
- Underwear, including large, close fitting pants (to hold maternity pads), and nursing bras.
- Towels.
- Maternity pads or night-time sanitary pads. (Large disposable nappies may be better for 24 hours after the birth.)
- Breast pads (to absorb leaks of colostrum and milk).
- Tissues.
- Phone card/coins.
- Toiletries and cosmetics.
- Nappies for baby.
- Something to read.
- Notepaper, pens, stamps and envelopes.
- Pack of biscuits or other snacks.
- Fruit juice/mineral water.

Bag three
(to go home)

- Baby clothes.
- Clothes for you.

Your will need a car seat for the journey home.

questions Q&A answered

Q. **My midwife has told me that my baby is in a 'posterior' position. She said that this may make my labour longer and that I will probably get backache. What is a posterior position, and can I do something about it?**

A. **A posterior position is when your baby's back is lying against your back. This position probably does not matter right now, but later, when you go into labour, your baby has to turn all the way around to the front. Whilst in this position his or her head presses against your sacrum (lower back) and can cause backache. However, there are some things you can do before your baby is born which may help.**

From about 36 weeks you might want to try using leaning forward positions whenever you can. This may help your baby to turn so that her back is towards your front, before her head becomes lodged in your pelvis. (Ideally, if this is your first baby, the back should also be to your left side.)

Possible things you could do:
- keep your knees lower than your hips
- keep your back above your tummy.

So, whenever you relax in front of the television, lean forward over a beanbag or lie on your left side on the couch. Whilst driving you can put a small cushion under the back of your bottom. If you have a posture seat, with knee rests, use it as much as you can. These adjustments to your posture can encourage your baby to turn the right way.

Weeks 37–40 plu

UP TO THE BIRTH DAY

These last weeks may seem to go slowly. Don't think of your baby as being 'due' on a certain day — many babies are later than this.

● At any time after week 36 or so, your baby's head may move well down into the pelvis. This is called 'engagement' (see below). You may now feel it's easier to breathe as your uterus exerts less pressure on your diaphragm. This is why the sensation you get is called 'lightening'.

● You'll probably feel different movements this late in pregnancy, as there is so little room in the uterus for the baby. Movements are more likely to feel 'big' rather than a series of smaller kicks. Your baby quite naturally has sleep times and wakeful times, so a quiet period may mean no more than a longish nap. However, contact the hospital, the midwife or the doctor if you don't feel your baby moving for several hours.

● The baby's lungs are maturing all the time, and she practises light breathing movements.

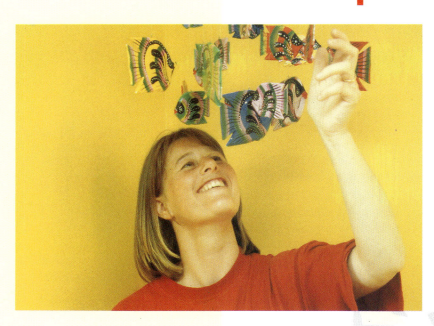

In the last two weeks of pregnancy, your baby may have a final growth spurt. At term, the average baby weighs between 3 and 4 kg (about 6 to 8 pounds) and measures about 50 to 60 cm (19½ to 23½ inches) long.

ENGAGEMENT

● Engagement of the head means that the largest diameter of the baby's head has passed the pelvic 'brim'. This means that the baby will fit through the pelvis and a normal birth should be possible. This happens most easily when the crown of the baby's head is coming first and the head is well 'curled' under. If this is not the case and the baby's head is in the posterior position (see page 31), or even if the 'brow' or 'face' is presenting, the head cannot fit into the pelvis.

● In many cases, and especially with posterior positions and in second or subsequent babies, when labour starts the baby's head will rotate and curl under with the power of the contractions. This means that the baby's head will fit into the pelvis and a normal birth will be possible. This is why in most cases it is wise to see what happens in labour (a 'trial of labour') rather than assume that there is disproportion — where the pelvis is too small for the baby's head, or its shape is not ideal — and have a planned Caesarean section. Sometimes, however, the head will not rotate or the pelvis will be definitely too small and a Caesarean section will be required.

ARE THESE 'REAL' CONTRACTIONS?

The uterus is formed of a network of strong muscle fibres, and contracts all the way through pregnancy. You may not be aware of this until later in your pregnancy (from 28 weeks onwards). The contractions can then be very noticeable. They are called **Braxton Hicks** contractions, and it can be easy to mistake them for labour.

You will feel your abdomen harden, and if you are in the bath, say, you will see it harden and remain tense for a number of seconds. Unlike labour contractions, Braxton Hicks contractions don't increase in length, intensity and frequency. They tend to be short, and come and go intermittently. Time them, and this will help you decide if it's the real thing or not.

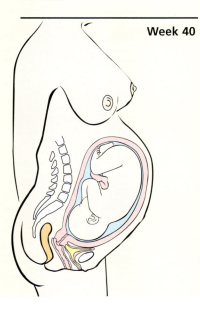

Week 40

questions Q&A answered

Q. My baby is breech. What does this mean?

A. It means that your baby is lying head-up in the uterus. His or her bottom is probably the part that will be born first — the presenting part. Occasionally, a foot is nearest the cervix (known as a footling breech).

Babies may lie with their legs bent at the knees, almost 'cross-legged', or with their legs straight up towards the face. This is known as a frank breech.

Q. How common is breech presentation?

A. At 30 weeks of pregnancy, about 20 per cent of babies are in the breech position. By term, the figure is down to three per cent. Many babies move into a head-down (vertex) position by themselves.

Q. What does this mean?

A. Babies who are still breech by about 37 weeks of pregnancy may not turn by themselves. Some doctors will carry out a manoeuvre called external cephalic version (ECV) to try to get them to turn. ECV is not usually done before 37 weeks/term.

Q. Will I need a Caesarean section?

A. Not necessarily. Some obstetricians prefer to deliver breech babies with a Caesarean section but many are born vaginally. Talk it over with your midwife and the consultant.

Q. Why am I more likely to need a Caesarean section?

A. The largest part of a baby is the head, and if the head is too large for the mother's pelvis, then it will not pass through. If the baby is coming head first then the problem will become obvious during labour. However, if the baby is breech, then the baby's bottom, which is smaller than its head, might pass through the pelvis and it will be more difficult to know if the head will fit safely through and not be damaged. Obstetricians are therefore reluctant to advise a 'trial of labour' if they have any concern at all that the baby's head will fit.

Antenatal care

WHERE AND WHAT TO EXPECT

Your antenatal care aims to check that you and your baby are well, and to pick up any problems before they become serious.

Where?

You'll probably have between 8 and 15 appointments. A few may be at the hospital antenatal clinic, but most of them will take place in the midwives' or GP's clinic, or at home.

What to expect

The booking appointment is the first major appointment, usually at about 8 to 12 weeks. You'll be asked a lot of questions to get a good picture of your health, and you'll be asked where you want to have your baby, so that a place can be booked for you (see page 47). You can change your mind later.

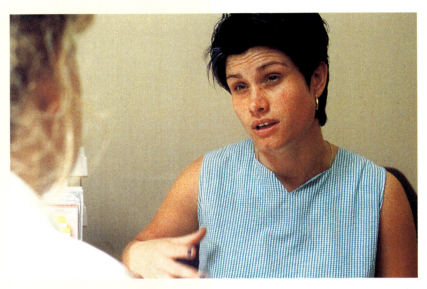

You can also ask questions yourself. This is an important chance for you to find out what you want to know. (See page 64 for information about antenatal classes.)

YOUR RECORDS

Your notes are the written record of your antenatal care. They have information about any previous pregnancies, and letters from any of the health professionals involved in your care. The results of any tests are also included.

You may carry your own notes, or they may be held at the doctor's, midwives' or hospital clinic. Instead of notes, you may look after the shared care card. This is a smaller version of your notes, containing the basic information about you and your pregnancy. Each time you have an antenatal appointment, the health professional you see records observations on the card, and signs it.

Take your notes/card with you if you go away from home for any length of time, in case you need to consult a doctor or a midwife. You are entitled to see a full copy of your notes at any time, before or after birth.

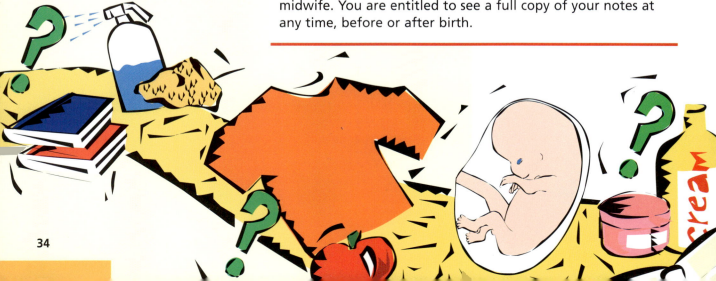

WORDS YOU MAY COME ACROSS

Here are some of the more common words you may come across when you read your notes, or overhear people talking:

ABORTION:
any pregnancy that ended before 24 weeks. A miscarriage is sometimes termed a 'spontaneous abortion'.

AFP:
alphafetoprotein. A substance present in the blood of pregnant women. Levels apparently higher or lower than normal may indicate the need for further tests (see pages 41–43).

ALB:
albumin, a protein substance. Your urine is tested for albumin, as it can be a sign of pre-eclampsia (see pages 55–56).

AMNIOTIC FLUID:
sometimes known as liquor (pronounced 'lye-kwor'). The fluid surrounding the baby in the uterus.

ANTENATAL:
before the birth.

APH:
antepartum haemorrhage — bleeding before birth.

BR:
breech presentation. A baby who is lying bottom or feet down in the uterus (the position of most babies until later pregnancy).

CEPH:
cephalic. The position of a baby who is lying head down in the uterus.

DIAPHRAGM:
muscle which lies across the top of the stomach, under the lungs (active in pushing baby out).

ECTOPIC PREGNANCY:
a pregnancy which develops somewhere other than the uterus, usually in the fallopian tube. The pregnancy must be terminated, as it is dangerous to the mother.

EDD:
expected date of delivery.

ENG:
engaged. Means that the largest diameter of the baby's head has passed the pelvic 'brim'.

EPISIOTOMY:
a cut made in the perineum (the skin between the vagina and the anus) to enable the baby to be born more quickly (see page 81).

FETUS:
medical term for the baby before it is born, ie when still in the uterus.

FH:
fetal heart. You may see 'FH heard' or 'FHH' on your notes. It means your baby's heartbeat has been heard.

FM:
fetal movement. You may see 'FM felt' or 'FMF' on your notes. It means your baby has been felt to move.

FUNDUS:
the top of the uterus. The fundal height is the length between the top of the uterus and the pubic bone. This helps date the pregnancy and assess the growth of the baby.

Hb:
haemoglobin. An indication of iron levels in the blood. If this is too low, this may indicate anaemia.

HYPERTENSION:
high blood pressure.

HYPOTENSION:
low blood pressure.

LIE:
the position of the baby in the uterus. You may see 'Long Lie' or 'LL' which

means longitudinal lie (the baby is straight up and down in the uterus).

MULTIGRAVIDA:
a woman who has had at least one pregnancy.

MULTIPARA:
sometimes called 'multip'. A woman who has given birth at least once before. A 'grand multipara' is a woman who has had at least four babies.

NAD:
'nothing abnormal detected', written when the doctor or midwife finds no problems.

OCCIPITO ANTERIOR:
the back of the baby's head is towards your front. You may see LOA or ROA on your notes, which mean 'left (or right) occipito anterior'. This describes whether the back of the head is towards the left or the right. LOA is usually the best position for a shorter labour and an easier birth.

OCCIPITO POSTERIOR:
the back of the baby's head is towards your back. LOP and ROP describe the position as left or right.

OEDEMA:
fluid retention, which causes swelling in your ankles, fingers and elsewhere.

PALPATION:
when the midwife or doctor feels the baby by moving their hands over your abdomen.

PERINEUM:
the area of skin between the vagina and the anus.

PIH:
pregnancy-induced hypertension (see page 39).

PLACENTA PRAEVIA:
when the placenta is low down. Sometimes it covers the cervix and blocks the baby's exit.

POSTNATAL:
after the birth.

PRESENTATION:
the position of the baby, with reference to the 'presenting part', that is the body part which will be born first (usually the vertex, or the back of the head).

PRE-TERM:
born before 37 weeks of pregnancy.

PRIMIGRAVIDA:
a woman pregnant for the first time.

PRIMIPARA:
sometimes called 'prim' or a 'primip' — a woman giving birth for the first time.

QUICKENING:
the first movements of the baby you can feel (see page 22).

Rh:
Rhesus (see page 40).

SUTURE:
the spaces between the bones in the baby's head.

TERM:
40 weeks (or thereabouts) from the first day of the last menstrual period.

VE:
vaginal examination.

VENTOUSE:
vacuum extraction (see pages 80–81).

VX:
vertex. The crown of the baby's head.

PEOPLE YOU'LL MEET

Caring for you and your baby

At the hospital, during antenatal care and if you plan to have your baby there, you may meet several different health professionals and others. Here's who they are, and what they do:

midwife — qualified in the care of mothers and babies during normal pregnancy and childbirth, and in the early days after the birth. Midwives are trained to recognise potential problems. There are hospital midwives, and community midwives who work outside the hospital. Community midwives may visit you at home before the birth, and will certainly visit after the birth.

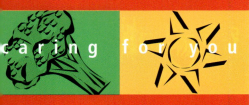

obstetrician — a specialist doctor in pregnancy and childbirth. You may see an obstetrician, or another qualified doctor who is training in obstetrics, if there is a problem with your pregnancy or birth, and maybe if everything is okay, too.

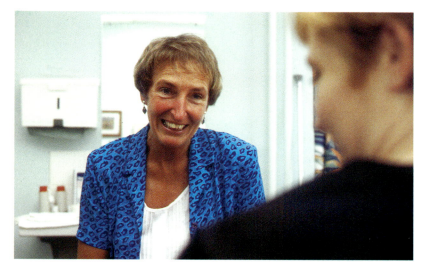

GP/family doctor — a doctor, who may also have an additional qualification in obstetrics. You can change your maternity care to a GP with this qualification, if you prefer. You may also see a GP Registrar, a qualified doctor gaining experience in general practice.

health visitor — a nurse who has undertaken extra training in child development and health promotion and who works in the community, either with a GP or according to a specific area. She or he gives support and advice to mothers and their children under five. This is your main source of information on child health and development shortly after the birth. You can visit your health visitor at the baby clinic, and he or she may come to meet you for the first time while you are still pregnant.

social worker — can help with advice and information on state benefits, and on housing difficulties, child care problems and so on.

dietitian — ask for advice if you have special dietary needs, whether connected with your pregnancy or not.

obstetric physiotherapist — may help you with postnatal exercises and possibly antenatal exercises, too. May be at parentcraft classes (see page 64).

paediatrician — a doctor who specialises in babies and children. If there are any worries about your baby's health, a paediatrician may be present at the birth. A paediatrician may also check your baby over before you go home from hospital.

radiographer — a technician who operates the ultrasound scanning equipment (see page 44).

radiologist — a doctor who specialises in ultrasound and X-rays.

Q. Will I be asked about how I plan to feed my baby?

A. You will be given a chance to discuss your feeding choice with your midwife or health visitor. You will be told about the health benefits of breastfeeding for you and your baby. This is not to press you to breastfeed, but to make sure you have all the information you need to make your choice.

Almost all maternity hospitals in Scotland are taking part in the UNICEF UK Baby Friendly Initiative. This international initiative aims to ensure mothers make an informed choice about how to feed their babies, and that hospitals and clinics use practices or routines which support mothers in their feeding choices.

A breastfeeding policy is usually on display.

Health benefits of breastfeeding to you and your baby

Breastfeeding protects your baby's health, not just now, but later on. Research shows that the benefits can last into toddlerhood and childhood. Breast milk builds immunity to infection, and aids the proper development of the brain. Breastfeeding reduces the risk of:

- gastro-enteritis — vomiting and diarrhoea
- ear infections
- wheeze when breathing/asthma
- eczema, where this ru in the family
- developing diabetes i childhood
- urinary infections
- chest infections.

Breast milk has a special for pre-term babies who are vulnerable to some v dangerous conditions an infections.

Mothers who breastfeed have a reduced risk of:

- ovarian cancer
- pre-menopausal brea cancer.

The table below shows how breastfeeding can be supported. Your midwife will discuss the points with you while you are pregnant, so that you know what to expect.

Supporting your choice to breastfeed: how it's done

What to expect	Why it's done
Skin to skin contact	● Keeps your baby warm ● Stabilises his breathing and his heartbea ● Helps you and your baby bond
Early first feed	● Your baby gets colostrum, rich in antibodies to help him fight infection, a help his first bowel movements
*Rooming in	● Helps you and your baby get to know ea other ● Makes baby-led feeding easier ● You and your baby sleep longer when you're together
Positioning and attachment	● Correct positioning and attachment help effective feeding, and help avoid sore nipples and other problems
Avoiding bottles and teats	● These may interfere with the way your b suckles at the breast and spoil his appeti for breastfeeds
Baby-led feeding	● Allows your baby to feed according to h hunger or thirst ● Helps your milk supply meet your baby's needs

*Note: rooming in simply means you and your baby are together in the same r

Many mothers find it's helpful to **write down their questions**, and then to read them at the appointment. No one will mind if you do this — health professionals know that it can be difficult to remember all you want to ask.

You may prefer to **talk after your examination** — even if the health professional says 'Anything you'd like to ask?' during it. Lying down is not the best position to talk! Just say, 'Yes, I have one or two things, can I ask them afterwards?'

If there's anything you don't understand, ask. You're bound to find things in your notes that puzzle you. Never worry that your question might sound trivial or make you appear silly. Doctors and midwives know it's important to have as much information as you want. You'll find a guide to some of the terms you may come across on pages 35–36.

Students may observe an antenatal appointment or your labour and birth, and in some cases, may treat you, under careful supervision. You should always be asked permission. If you prefer not to have a student observing or treating you, just say no. The same applies to research projects. You should always be asked for permission if researchers want to include you and your experience in their studies. Again, you can say no if you prefer.

CHECKS AND TESTS DURING PREGNANCY

Always ask the reason for tests — they may be routine and straightforward to the health professionals carrying them out, but not to you. Some tests are not offered to all women — talk to your midwife or doctor about these tests (see below).

Routine tests
Blood tests

You'll probably be offered at least one blood test in pregnancy, taken at your first appointment. This can:

- measure your haemoglobin (full blood count), which is a way of assessing the level of iron in your blood. If it is low it indicates you could be anaemic, and you may be offered iron tablets or other appropriate treatments.

- identify your blood group (A, B, O or AB)

- see whether you are Rhesus positive or negative (see page 40)

- check your levels of immunity to Rubella (German measles). Most women have been immunised, but if necessary you can be offered immunisation after the birth.

- check for syphilis. This is a sexually acquired infection. It is now rare, but if undetected it can seriously damage your health and that of your baby by causing developmental difficulties. Effective treatment (course of antibiotics) is available if the test result is positive.

- check for hepatitis B, a viral infection which causes liver disease and can be transmitted to your baby during or just after delivery. If you test positive, your baby will receive a complete course of a very effective vaccine and injections of antibodies called immunoglobin immediately after birth.

- check for Human Immunodeficiency Virus (HIV), the virus that causes Acquired Immunodeficiency Syndrome (AIDS). Infected pregnant women can pass HIV to their babies during pregnancy, childbirth and also through breastfeeding. If your HIV result is positive, advice and treatment under the guidance of specialists will be offered. Such interventions include treatment with special drugs and advice about the best type of delivery and method of feeding your baby to reduce the chance of the baby also getting the infection.

All these tests will be carried out unless you request otherwise. If you have any questions or concerns about these tests, please ask at your next clinic visit or contact your midwife.

Usually, a blood test means no more than taking a little blood from a vein in your arm. The blood is drawn up through a needle into a syringe. A blood test shouldn't be painful, though there may be slight bruising for a day or so afterwards.

Blood pressure

Your blood pressure is checked at most appointments. This is to make sure you have no signs of **pre-eclampsia**, or **pregnancy-induced hypertension** (see pages 55–56). The midwife or doctor wraps a fabric band around your arm and inflates it with a small pump. The cuff is linked to a blood pressure measure. As the cuff deflates, the midwife or doctor uses a stethoscope to listen to changes of your pulse.

A high reading may give cause for concern, so some health professionals will do the test again, 10 or 20 minutes later, to make doubly sure.

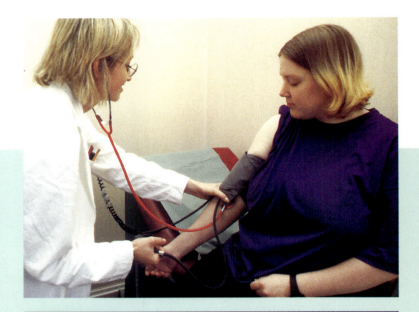

Urine

Your urine will be tested for **protein** and **sugar.** (A special strip is dipped into a sample which you either bring with you or produce at the appointment.) Some women develop a particular sort of diabetes that occurs in pregnancy — **gestational diabetes**. This might first show as sugar in the urine. Protein might indicate pre-eclampsia. Infections of the kidney and bladder might show up here, too.

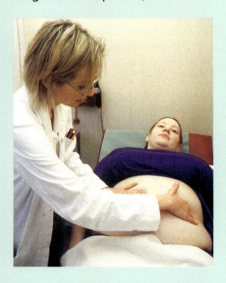

Abdomen

Your abdomen will be **palpated** at each visit. This means the doctor or midwife feels the way your baby is lying, and its size, and the height of your uterus, by moving her hands around the outside of your abdomen.

questions Q&A answered

Q. **I have Rhesus negative blood, and I have been told I need injections to prevent my baby from being harmed. Can you explain?**

A. **Most people (80 per cent) have Rhesus positive blood (written in notes as Rh+ or Rh+ve). If you have Rhesus negative blood, and the father of your baby has Rhesus negative blood, too, there's no problem because your baby will have the same type. If you have Rhesus negative blood and the father is Rhesus positive, then your baby could be positive, which might cause a problem.**

In a first pregnancy your bloodstream and your baby's don't usually meet until the birth. Then they may come into contact when the placenta is delivered. As a result, in a second or subsequent pregnancy, your blood will produce antibodies which could cause a serious blood disorder in your baby. To avoid this, you will be offered injections of Anti-D gammaglobulin after your pregnancy, or during it if you have any bleeding. In some areas, Rhesus negative women may be offered injections during pregnancy whether or not there has been bleeding.

Screening and diagnostic tests in pregnancy

Some mothers may be offered tests which aren't appropriate for everyone. You can choose whether or not to have them, and you may want to discuss this with your midwife or doctor.

- A **screening test** aims to tell you if there is a risk that you or your baby may have a problem.

- A **diagnostic** test is done to show whether a problem actually exists. Many tests are useful, and some are very important, but no test is perfect — it may miss the thing it is designed to look for, (a 'false negative'), or it may seem to show something that isn't there (a 'false positive').

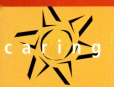
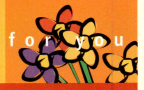

caring for you

Screening tests

Double test

After 15 weeks of pregnancy, you may be offered a blood test called a **double test**. It measures the amount of two substances, AFP and HCG. From the results, the chance of Down's Syndrome, spina bifida or other neutral tube defects (NTDs) is calculated. It's a screening test, and does not diagnose anything.

A higher or lower level than normal of AFP and/or HCG can mean an increased risk of the baby having these conditions. The testers also need to know both the number of weeks you are pregnant and your age to calculate the chance for Down's syndrome and for NTDs.

You should receive the results within 10 days, and you are told what chance you have of having a baby with a particular condition.

With chromosomal disorders such as Down's syndrome (see later), the result may be expressed as a 'one in something' chance. So, if you are told your result is a 'one in 400', it means your baby has a 1 in 400 chance of being affected by the disability. That is, for every 400 pregnancies with the same result, 399 are likely to be normal.

Diagnostic tests

Depending on the results of screening tests, you may be offered a further test, such as **amniocentesis**, or **ultrasound**, which aim to diagnose any problem. In most cases, these further tests show your baby is healthy. If not, then you will be offered counselling to help you decide what to do.

Chorionic villus sampling (CVS) and amniocentesis (see over) check for chromosomal abnormalities, principally Down's syndrome.

These tests are usually offered only to women who have a higher chance of having a baby with a disability because there is a chance that the test may cause a miscarriage. An older mother, for example, is more likely to have a baby with Down's syndrome. A test may also be offered to a mother who has had a previous pregnancy affected by one of these abnormalities.

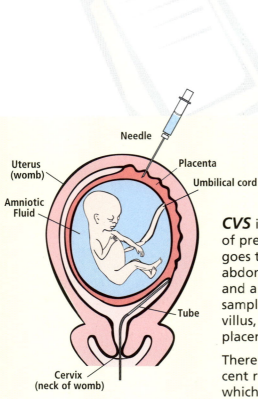

Needle
Uterus (womb)
Placenta
Umbilical cord
Amniotic Fluid
Tube
Cervix (neck of womb)

CVS is done after 10 weeks of pregnancy. A fine tube goes through your cervix or abdomen into the womb, and a syringe removes a sample of the chorionic villus, the tissue forming the placenta.

There is a two to four per cent risk of miscarriage, which will be discussed with you. Results take between 7 and 10 days.

Amniocentesis is done later, after 14 weeks. The syringe takes a sample of the amniotic fluid, after a needle is inserted into the uterus, through the abdomen.

There is a one per cent risk of miscarriage, which will be discussed with you, and results can take from 10 days to a few weeks.

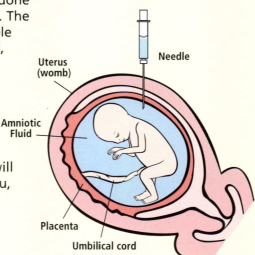

Uterus (womb)
Needle
Amniotic Fluid
Placenta
Umbilical cord

Ultrasound scanning will be used if you have CVS or amniocentesis, so that the doctor can see the exact position of the baby and the placenta. Scans are also sometimes used to detect some abnormalities. See page 44 for more information about ultrasound scanning.

Other tests you may have

You may be offered a blood test to check for past or present infection with the **cytomegalovirus (CM** virus), and for **toxoplasmosis** (see page 14).

All areas offer testing for **cystic fibrosis** after birth (see page 88). However in some areas there may be a simple test to check if you are a carrier of the disease. This test involves giving you a mouthwash, to collect cells from the lining of your mouth. Tell the midwife or doctor if you have a family history of this condition.

Antenatal screening and diagnosis is an area where change takes place all the time. Tests that were once offered in only a few parts of the country while their effects were being studied have become more widely available. So there may be tests on offer in your area which we haven't covered here. Before you agree to any test, you should be told how effective and reliable a test is, and if there are any side-effects.

Note: if you have Rhesus negative blood, you will be advised to have an anti-D injection after CVS and after amniocentesis.

Is there a problem?

When tests show there could be a problem, you need more information, and support.

- It's important to know what the test result shows, whether it's conclusive or not, and whether you need to make any decisions about labour or birth, or the future of your pregnancy.

- You may need time to consider your options. There are support groups that can help you with these difficult decisions (see **Further help**) and you can ask to talk with a midwife or a health visitor, as well as a doctor. If the tests indicate a disability, you may want to talk to parents who have a child with a similar condition, to get information about it. No one should try to influence you in any way; the decision has to be yours, and your partner's.

Q. I have been advised to have an amniocentesis. But I don't want to have one. Am I right?

A. Only you can decide. There is a small risk of miscarriage with amniocentesis, and you may want to compare that with the risk of having a baby with an abnormality. Discuss the comparative risks with your doctor. Or, you may not want to have a termination of pregnancy under any circumstances, and if this is the case, then there is no real reason to have an amniocentesis — though some parents want to know if their child will have a disability in order to prepare themselves for it. In any event, it is your right to decide whether or not you accept the offer of a test.

'My greatest fear was having a baby with some sort of disability, and I knew I was at a higher risk of a baby with Down's syndrome because of my age. When the amniocentesis came back and it was negative, I felt I could relax, and tell people about the pregnancy at last.'

'There is a downside to antenatal tests. My AFP test came back with a query, and I needed further investigation to rule out spina bifida. I was told there was probably nothing to worry about, but of course I did. Even when I was given the "all clear" I still worried, in case they had missed something. I think it increased my anxiety, for nothing.'

Ultrasound

SCANNING YOUR BABY DURING PREGNANCY

An ultrasound scan uses high-frequency soundwaves which bounce off solid objects. It creates a picture on a screen of your baby, the uterus, the placenta and the baby's organs. You may be offered one or more ultrasound scans.

Scans can give you and the doctor and midwife information about your baby's growth and development. They can tell you:

- your baby's size. This helps establish the dates of your pregnancy, and to ensure your baby is growing as expected

- the way your baby is lying in the uterus, which might be important at the end of pregnancy

- if twins or more are present

- the development of your baby's organs, and bones (including the spine).

They can also show:

- some abnormalities

- the exact position of the baby and placenta, to allow amniocentesis and/or CVS (see pages 41–42 for details of these procedures)

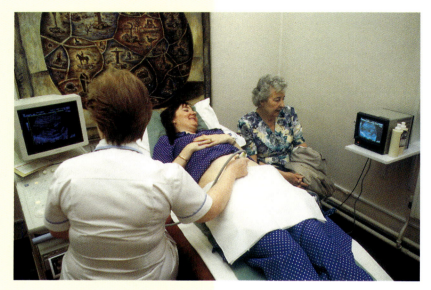

- where the placenta is lying — in late pregnancy, a low-lying placenta might cause severe bleeding, and could prevent the baby from being born vaginally (which means you'd need a Caesarean section).

When the scan is offered may differ according to local policies. For example, most units offer a scan at around 12 weeks, and again later if a problem arises. If you don't wish to have any scans, or fewer than the number offered, then of course you don't have to have them.

Preparing for a scan

For a scan in early pregnancy, you'll be asked to fill your bladder first by drinking lots of water. The fullness in your bladder then pushes the uterus upwards, and this helps the radiographer get a better picture. This is a bit uncomfortable for you, as you will be dying to use the toilet for a while!

How it's done

You lie down on a flat couch, and the doctor or radiographer stands or sits next to you. You need to roll down your lower clothing, and lift up your top, so your tummy is exposed. The radiographer or doctor spreads some cold gel on your abdomen. Then a hand-held microphone-like instrument called a transducer is rolled over your abdomen. This picks up a picture of everything underneath it, and transmits it to a screen where it appears as a picture. The whole process is painless.

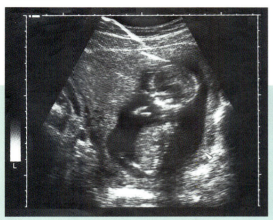

Is ultrasound safe? Most obstetricians feel there is no good evidence that ultrasound harms your baby's health or development, though it's difficult to show conclusive proof of safety. There is little evidence to show that routine scanning reduces the number of pregnancies with problems or the number of babies suffering from slow growth.

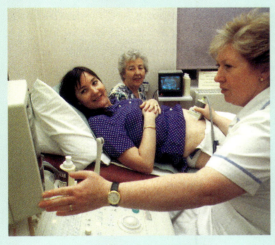

Many parents themselves report feeling reassured when a scan shows no problems. However, in the few cases where ultrasound reveals an unexpected problem, the information gained may help you and your doctors to reach a decision about whether or not to continue with the pregnancy.

questions Q&A answered

Q. Can the scan also show whether I am having a girl or a boy?

A. Sometimes. If you want to know, just ask. You won't be told unless you want to be. You do need to bear in mind that the picture may not be clear enough, or the baby may be lying in such a way that the genitals aren't visible. The answer you get may not be the correct one.

You may not actually recognise a baby when you see the image on the screen. But the radiographer or radiologist carrying out the scan can trace the outline of your baby's body, and point out the placenta and indicate the major body organs. You will probably be able to see your baby's heart beating, and to see what position he is lying in. It may be possible for you to take away a photograph of the scanned image. You may be charged a small fee for this.

Q. Can my partner be with me when I have the scan?

A. Usually, yes. Or, take someone else with you if you prefer. Check before you have the scan that this is acceptable; very few places now discourage a companion.

'The first time I saw my baby on the screen was the first time I really felt pregnant — it was a wonderful moment.'

'I didn't want to have a scan. I wasn't convinced it was necessary — and though everyone just assumed I would have one, no one criticised me for saying no.'

Your choices and how to make them

WHERE AND HOW TO HAVE YOUR BABY

Talk over the choices available with a midwife, your family doctor, your partner, with other mothers you know who have had babies in your area, and with local childbirth organisations.

The choice of places for your labour and birth includes:

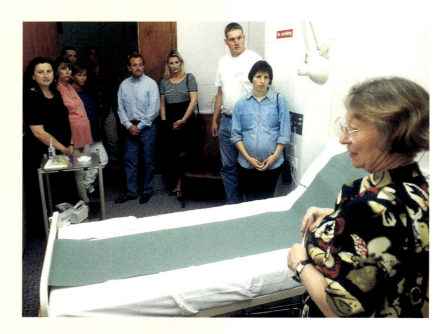

- **hospital, in a consultant-led unit** (though midwives carry out most of the care). There may be more than one unit in your area. A consultant-led unit is usually chosen if you expect to need a doctor's help. Some women who have no problems still feel reassured by having specialist medical care on hand

- **hospital, in a midwife-led unit** (see page 47), if available in your area

- **domino birth**. The community midwife visits you in early labour, goes with you to hospital for the birth and may return home with you later. In some areas, there are variations on this.

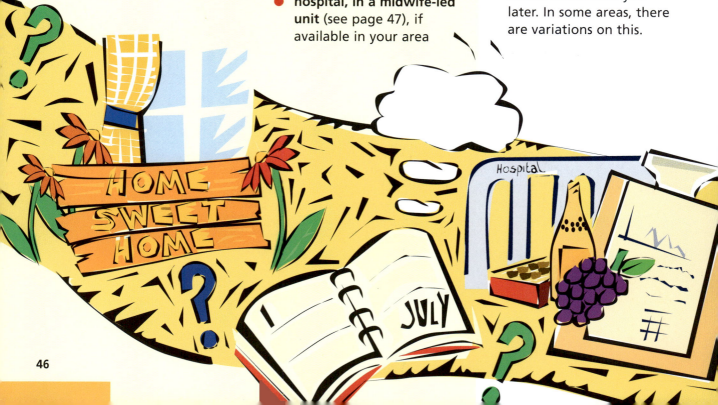

HOME SWEET HOME

Hospital

JULY

- **at home.** There is no evidence that a planned home birth is less safe than anywhere else for women who are not expected to have problems with pregnancy or birth. If you live in an isolated area, some way from a hospital, you may need to reconsider a decision to have a home birth.

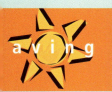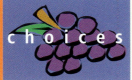

a v i n g   c h o i c e s

You're usually asked to **'book' your place of birth** near the beginning of pregnancy, but you don't have to stick with your original decision though it is important that your doctor and midwife both know your plan. Once your family doctor knows you are pregnant, a midwife may come to your home to book you, or else you'll be offered an appointment at the hospital of your choice.

- Midwives care for all women, with medical help if needed. The doctor's role is to care for the small number of women and babies who need medical care.

- Some units in hospitals are known as **midwife-led units**, which means the midwives are responsible for running the whole unit. Generally, a midwife-led unit cares for women expecting a normal birth. For this reason, mothers expecting to need a doctor's involvement will not be encouraged to book there.

- You may be introduced to your 'named midwife' — a midwife you will see during your antenatal care and when you return home after your baby is born. In other areas, you may meet members of a team of midwives.

Independent midwives usually offer their services to women for a fee. Sometimes they charge according to your ability to pay. Increasingly, independent midwives work alongside their health service colleagues. You can still give birth at home or in hospital, as you wish. There are a few independent midwives in Scotland. For more information, see **Further help.**

'I knew the only place I would really feel comfortable and relaxed was at home. Everything's going well, and I have met most of the midwives who are likely to deliver me — that's important.'

'I prefer the idea of hospital, where there are staff and equipment immediately at hand, in case something goes wrong. We are going to visit the delivery suite, as we'd both like to know what to expect beforehand.'

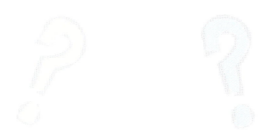

Q. I would like a home birth, but I have been told home births aren't available in my area.

A. Home births may be rare in your area but you can still choose this if you wish. Book it with your community midwife at your local maternity unit. The supervisor of midwives there should then arrange for antenatal care for you, and make sure you have midwifery care for birth and afterwards. If you have any problems you can contact the supervisor of midwives direct.

WHAT SORT OF BIRTH IS RIGHT FOR YOU?

Your midwife may ask you during pregnancy if you would like to make a **birth plan.** This means that your choices are written down, after a full discussion, and after you feel you have the information on which to base your choices.

The birth plan then goes into your notes, with a copy for you to keep. Your choices are important guidelines and reminders, but you can still change your mind.

These are some of the issues you may want to consider:

- is it important for you to avoid induction or acceleration of labour? (See page 75.)

- who will be your birth companion(s)?

- do you want to use a birthing pool or bath for labour and/or birth?

- how do you want your baby's heart rate to be monitored? (See page 74.)

- do you want to be free to move into different positions during labour and delivery?

- what about pain relief? (See pages 50–51.)

- do you prefer an unaided 'physiological' third stage or an 'actively managed' third stage? (See pages 82–83.)

- are you planning to breastfeed or bottle feed? (Don't feel you have to make up your mind right away — some women aren't sure at this stage.)

- (for hospital birth) when do you think you might like to return home after the birth?

- what about Vitamin K? Most maternity units offer an injection of Vitamin K to your baby shortly after birth. This is to prevent a rare disease in newborn babies called haemorrhagic disease of the newborn which can cause bleeding inside the baby in the first few days of life. (See page 89 for further information.)

When your baby is born you will be asked if you want your baby to have the Vitamin K supplement. So, during pregnancy you will need to consider this and you may want to ask your midwife, health visitor or doctor for further information.

Water birth

Labouring in water can help you relax, and women often report that it helps with the pain of contractions. Far more women use the bath for labour than actually give birth to their babies in it.

You can discuss the possibility of delivering your baby in the water with the midwife or midwives who will be caring for you (if you plan a home birth) or with the antenatal clinic and the labour ward midwife (if you plan to go to hospital).

If you would like to stay in the water for a long time, it's better to use a large pool with plenty of room for you to change positions, and with room all round it. Then the midwife can examine you from all sides if necessary, and help the baby out. The water needs to be kept warm. Some hospitals have a birthing pool, or a large bath they use for labour. You can hire a special pool for use at home (see 'Pregnancy and Maternity Services' in the **Further help** section at the back of this book).

Some units do not permit staff to attend water births or will not allow delivery under water in their facility.

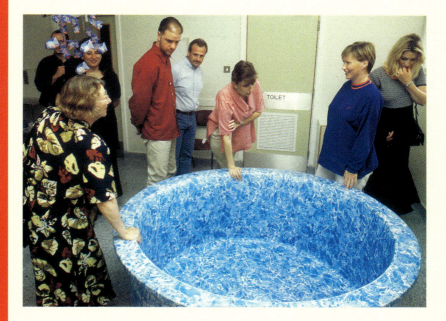

Is water birth safe? Many questions have been raised about water birth safety, and there may be concerns about cross-infection. Opinions differ amongst midwives and obstetricians — some are doubtful, others feel that with the right care, water birth is a safe option.

In the end, the choice is yours. But if you are having your baby in a hospital which has no proper facilities for water birth, or whose staff do not feel confident with water birth, you may want to think about having your baby elsewhere.

Who will be with you at the birth?

Who would you like to give you support and encouragement when you're in labour? Your partner may be the obvious choice, if you have one, but it doesn't have to be. It can be a friend.

There's some evidence that having another person with you, instead of, or as well as, your partner, is helpful, and can shorten your labour. Some women have a close friend, a relative, or their antenatal teacher. A good relationship with the professional carers is important to your whole labour — but having a companion you know already may be important, too.

PAIN RELIEF IN LABOUR

Discuss your choice of pain relief before you go into labour. Your midwife or doctor will tell you what's available. You'll be able to talk about your choices in antenatal classes, too.

You may wish to use self-help forms of pain relief or to have pain-relieving drugs of some type.

Non-chemical pain relief

Most antenatal classes teach breathing awareness, as a way of coping with the pain of contractions. The emphasis is on breathing as a way of relaxation, which helps you cope with the pain.

Relaxation doesn't take away pain, but it can prevent pain becoming stronger, because tension increases pain levels. The main aim is to help you to be able to cope with the pain and not be overwhelmed by it. Then you will be fully conscious, and in as much control of your labour as you want to be. There is research to show that when women are relaxed, they release the body's own hormone-like pain-relievers — endorphins.

It is important to some women to avoid drugs in labour, as all drug-based methods have some disadvantages to mother or baby or both. You may want to rely on yourself, with the support and encouragement of those around you. There are no disadvantages to breathing and relaxation, but sometimes they may not work if your labour is long, complicated, or just too painful for you.

Other various non-drug pain relief includes *homoeopathy*, *hypnosis*, *acupuncture* and *acupressure*. You need to see a practitioner in these methods first. *Lying in water* can also help (see page 49), as can *massage*.

TENS — stands for **Transcutaneous Electrical Nerve Stimulation**. It is a form of pain relief provided by a small box wired to electrodes which fix on your skin, and which give out a slight electrical charge. It can be effective in relieving pain, and it is safe for you and your baby. If you want to use this, ask the hospital if you can hire or borrow a TENS machine so that you can start to use it as soon as labour begins.

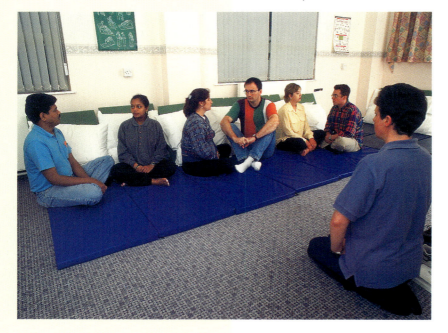

Entonox — **sometimes known as 'laughing gas', or 'gas and air'. This is the brand name for the mix of 50 per cent nitrous oxide, and 50 per cent oxygen. The gas comes in a cylinder, attached to a tube and a mask which you place on your face. There may be a mouthpiece you can use instead. At the start of a contraction, begin taking deep breaths of gas.**

Effects: the effects start about 15 or 20 seconds after you first breathe it in. If it works for you, it takes the 'edge' off the peak of the pain and this relief lasts until the end of the contraction. You can't overdose on Entonox. This is because you become drowsy as you use it, and your hand holding the mask or mouthpiece just falls away as you drop off, preventing you from breathing in any more. Your body also expels this gas quickly.

Babies appear not to be affected; very little Entonox reaches them.

Diamorphine and pethidine — **drugs which are related to morphine and are commonly given in labour. They are given by injection and the dose can be varied.**

Effects: they take around 15 minutes to work and last for two to four hours. You may feel sleepy and slightly 'out of it', as if the pain is there but you're not experiencing it. Some women feel this distancing effect as 'being out of control'. Some women feel sick with these drugs and an anti-sickness medicine is usually given at the same time.

Pethidine can affect the baby's breathing at birth. The baby may be sleepier and less interested in feeding for two or three days afterwards. If your baby's breathing is poor as a result of pethidine a drug can be given to treat this. The effect on breathing is more likely if the injection is given too close to the birth, and you may be advised not to have it for this reason. If pethidine is given four or more hours before birth, the effects have a better chance to wear off in the mother. The effects will remain in the baby for longer, say up to 48 hours, after birth.

Epidural anaesthesia — **an anaesthetic drug is injected into the epidural space at the side of the spinal cord. You may be asked to curl up on your side while the anaesthetist inserts the epidural, or you may be able to sit up, leaning forward over a pillow. A fine plastic tube — a catheter — is left in so that more anaesthetic can be given if needed. You're usually given a drip to help maintain normal blood pressure (low blood pressure can be a side-effect). It is likely that the baby's heartbeat will be continually monitored.**

Effects: total pain relief for most women (although for a few they may only get relief down one side). You may have no feeling at all in the lower half of your body, which may make it harder for you to push in second stage. This numbness will last for some hours. It will be less likely that you will be able to adopt kneeling or squatting positions for labour or delivery.

Just occasionally, you may have a bad headache for some days after the birth, and some mothers may get backache.

Forceps delivery may be more common because you can lose the urge to push. On the other hand, some doctors feel that having an epidural, especially for a long labour might increase the chances of a vaginal delivery, as the pain relief and relaxation some women experience with it allows labour to be augmented (see page 75) with syntocinon and to progress.

Are all forms of pain relief always available?

At home, the midwife can give you Entonox, and/or pethidine. In hospital you usually have all forms available, although in some units epidurals may not be available round the clock as there may be no anaesthetist there.

Changes to your body

MINOR PROBLEMS

Most women will experience some of these very common 'side-effects' of pregnancy — but you'd be very unlucky to have them all!

If you have persistent problems, see your doctor or you may like to try alternative remedies as prescribed by an expert.

FOOD CRAVINGS — very common at any stage in pregnancy. You may want odd food combinations, or get a liking for large quantities of something you haven't enjoyed before. As long as you continue to eat a healthy diet (see page 13) you don't need to worry.

BLEEDING GUMS/GINGIVITIS — you may find that your gums bleed more easily during pregnancy. Make sure you clean your teeth and gums thoroughly twice a day using a fluoride toothpaste. Remember dental treatment is free while you are pregnant and for a year after the birth of your child. It is a good idea to have your teeth and gums checked by your dentist.

HEARTBURN (INDIGESTION) — a burning sensation round the breastbone, caused by stomach juices and foods. It's more common in later pregnancy. Eat small amounts of food more often if you are affected by this. Take your time when you eat. Strong tea/coffee, pure fruit juice, spicy and fatty foods can cause heartburn.

CONSTIPATION — this is very common in pregnancy. Eat more fresh fruit and vegetables and more wholegrain breads and cereals, to increase your fibre intake. Drink more — a glass of water with every meal and in between.

THRUSH — a thick white vaginal discharge, accompanied by itching and soreness, also known as candidiasis. Your doctor can prescribe vaginal pessaries, tested as safe to use in pregnancy.

PASSING URINE OFTEN — this is normal, and caused by pregnancy hormones and the increasing compression of your bladder. Occasionally, there may be a urine infection. Mention it your midwife.

STRESS INCONTINENCE — the bladder leaks a little urine. This happens because the pelvic floor muscles are put under stress when you cough, sneeze or run. It happens especially in later pregnancy. Pelvic floor exercises (see pages 102–103) can help to strengthen the muscles. If necessary, wear a pad to keep you comfortable. Continue to do your exercises after the birth.

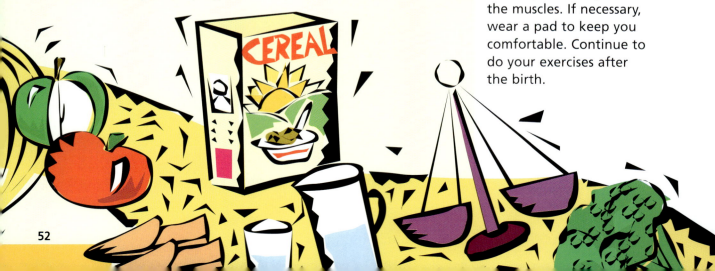

CYSTITIS — a urine infection causing a burning sensation on passing urine, and the feeling of needing to pass urine all the time. If persistent your doctor can treat this. Try drinking lots of water to help flush out the infection.

VARICOSE VEINS — swollen veins, usually in the legs but sometimes in the vulva (vaginal opening), too. They may cause aching and sometimes itching. Support tights or stockings can help. Don't stand for long periods, and rest with your legs up when you can. Always tell your midwife or doctor if you notice any hot, red or painful areas in your legs.

PILES OR HAEMORRHOIDS — these are varicose veins of the back passage, or anus. They are sometimes painful and itchy, and they can be made worse by constipation. Your doctor can treat them.

BACKACHE — flat shoes or shoes with a low heel will help. Sit and stand with your back straight, and shoulders dropped. Be careful about lifting heavy weights —

always bend at the knees to do so. There are some specific exercises that can help — ask your midwife, obstetric physiotherapist or antenatal teacher.

SWELLING OF THE ANKLES, FINGERS, FACE AND HANDS, or oedema, happens because the body holds more fluid in pregnancy. A certain amount of oedema is normal in later pregnancy, but more severe cases can indicate pre-eclampsia, if present with other signs (see pages 55–56).

Sometimes fluid collects in the wrists and produces a painful or tingling sensation in the fingers. This is called 'carpal tunnel syndrome'. Raising your hands above your head for several minutes may help to drain the fluid away. If it is very troublesome, speak to your midwife or GP. They can refer you to an obstetric physiotherapist who may give you lightweight splints to wear on your wrists. The condition usually goes away after the birth.

HOW MUCH WEIGHT IS GAINED IN PREGNANCY?

You can expect to gain between 9 and 16 kg (19 and 35 pounds) in weight during your pregnancy. The average is about 12.5 kg (28 pounds).

Your weight gain is made up like this:

- baby 2.5–4 kg (5–9 pounds)
- placenta 500–1000 g (1–2 pounds)
- amniotic fluid 1.5–2.5 kg (3–5 pounds)
- extra weight of uterus, breasts and energy stores of fat 2–5 kg (4–11 pounds)
- extra weight of blood 2–4 kg (4–9 pounds).

You may gain weight from the very start of pregnancy, mainly because of extra fluid and fluid retention. Many women put on very little in the last two to three weeks, or stop gaining altogether.

You'll be weighed at the start of the pregnancy, for future comparisons, but you may not be weighed at every antenatal appointment. This is because the information gained is not always useful, and weighing can make some women unnecessarily anxious.

Don't keep your worries to yourself. Most pregnancy problems aren't serious for you or your baby's health (although they may not seem so at the time). Your midwife or doctor will give you advice and reassurance about how to deal with most of the less serious discomforts of pregnancy.

If you need to talk to a midwife, call the antenatal clinic at the hospital where you plan to give birth. If you know someone by name, ask for that person. Or you can telephone your community midwife.

More serious problems

IS THERE SOMETHING WRONG?

You may need treatment, or careful observation, if there are signs of more serious problems in your pregnancy. These problems include:

Anaemia

This means you are lacking in iron, and/or folic acid, and/or Vitamin B12. The condition shows up in a blood test. Anaemia may be a result of illness, poor diet, severe sickness, or extra strain on your body such as when you are expecting twins. You will be given information on changing your diet, and you may be prescribed iron supplements.

Bleeding

You should get medical advice straight away if you notice you are bleeding from the vagina in pregnancy, or if you experience severe, abdominal pain. Sometimes, the placenta is lying so low it covers the cervix. It is more likely to bleed in this position. This condition — placenta

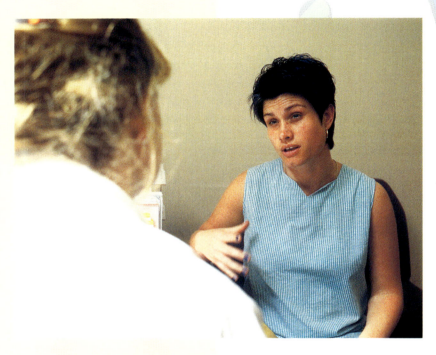

praevia — is uncommon and needs careful observation. Any bleeding from the vagina in pregnancy should be taken seriously. In later pregnancy it could be that the placenta is separating from the uterine wall. This could be life-threatening to you and your baby.

Not all instances of bleeding are serious — some women do bleed a little on and off all the way through pregnancy, for a variety of minor reasons.

Continued sickness

If you are unfortunate, the pregnancy sickness that usually goes at around

12 weeks persists into later pregnancy. Very severe cases, known as hyperemesis gravidarum, need hospital treatment.

Diabetes

Some women develop diabetes during pregnancy. The condition disappears after pregnancy, though some women do go on to develop diabetes later. The pregnancy may be affected, as the baby tends to get larger, and the diabetes will be monitored to make sure it remains under control.

High blood pressure

When blood pressure is very high it can be diagnosed as pregnancy-induced hypertension. If it's present with other symptoms it can be a sign of pre-eclampsia (see right and page 56). High blood pressure can affect the placenta.

Itching

Occasionally women develop a severe itching of the skin in pregnancy. This is usually no more than a highly irritating discomfort — but occasionally it can be the sign of a condition called obstetric cholestasis, which can affect the liver. See your doctor or midwife if your itch doesn't clear up, or if no treatment helps.

OTHER PROBLEMS

Separated symphysis pubis

This happens when the small joint (the symphysis pubis) at the front of the bony girdle of the pelvis opens up too far. It can happen in pregnancy or at birth. It can cause a lot of pain on walking or even standing. Physiotherapy can help, or a support belt worn across the pelvis to keep the joint together while it gets back to its normal pre-pregnancy state. (See also **Further help** at the back of this book.)

Separation of the long abdominal muscles

When this happens, the uterus needs extra support as the pregnancy progresses.

PRE-ECLAMPSIA

This condition occurs only in pregnancy, and affects one in every 10 pregnancies. Most cases are mild, but some (about one first pregnancy in every 100) are dangerous for the baby and the mother.

When a mother has severe pre-eclampsia or eclampsia, her labour may be induced, even though this might mean a pre-term delivery.

The condition is called 'pre' (before) eclampsia because if it is not treated or treated too late it can develop into eclampsia, a rare but serious complication characterised by convulsions. However, eclampsia is not the only serious complication of pre-eclampsia: affected women may also develop problems with the liver, lungs, kidneys, brain or blood clotting system. The signs of pre-eclampsia are:

- rising blood pressure in mid to late pregnancy
- protein present in the urine
- severe oedema (swelling), due to fluid retention, in the ankles, fingers, face
- headaches/visual disturbances
- severe pain just below the ribs
- poor growth in the baby.

'Do I have to go into hospital?'

Today, some conditions are observed and treated at home, perhaps by the GP or the community midwife. Sometimes, you can go into hospital for daycare only, returning home at night.

However, if you are at risk of bleeding, or of going into pre-term labour, hospital may be the best place for you, especially if your home is some distance away and you cannot get to hospital quickly in an emergency. Sometimes, pregnant women go into hospital because of severe sickness, or because they have a condition that needs to be watched.

Routine antenatal checking of your blood pressure and your urine in pregnancy is mainly to detect the development of pre-eclampsia.

The cause of pre-eclampsia and/or high blood pressure is not fully understood, and the links between the main signs are still very unclear. At least two of the main signs must be present before pre-eclampsia is diagnosed.

Note: In very serious cases of pre-eclampsia, the mother may feel very unwell. She may vomit, and have a very bad headache, visual disturbances and severe pain just below the ribs. Always report these symptoms to the midwife or doctor.

For more information see the **Further help** section.

Q. **My baby isn't growing very well. Is this serious?**

A. **It may be, but some babies are naturally small, and some catch up in later pregnancy. Your dates may be incorrect, so you may not be as far on in your pregnancy as you think. Most babies are born healthy. It's very difficult to diagnose accurately if a baby isn't growing well. Most small babies are born well and grow into normal healthy children.**

Some babies have intrauterine growth retardation (IUGR), which means they are smaller and lighter than most healthy babies at this stage of pregnancy. IUGR may happen because the placenta isn't nourishing the baby well, or perhaps because the baby has an underlying condition which is preventing growth. If the mother's diet is very poor, this can cause poor growth in the baby. Smoking also causes the baby to be less well-nourished, and therefore smaller. Occasionally, poor growth in the baby can be a sign of pre-eclampsia in the mother.

Very small babies are at a greater risk of pre-term birth and its hazards. They may have development problems that go on into childhood. Sometimes, the baby has a better chance of growing and surviving outside the uterus, and the doctor may advise you that the best option is to induce labour (see page 67).

If your baby isn't growing well, further investigations will be discussed with you. You may have more scans, for example, so that your baby's development can be measured more accurately.

Pregnancy & work

YOUR RIGHTS AND BENEFITS

You need to make decisions regarding your job. When can you leave before your baby is born? Do you plan to return after your baby, and if so, when?

Maternity leave

All pregnant employees with babies due on or after 6 April 2003 are able to take 26 weeks Ordinary Maternity Leave (OML). You can take OML regardless of how long you have worked for your employer and how many hours you work. If you have worked for your employer for

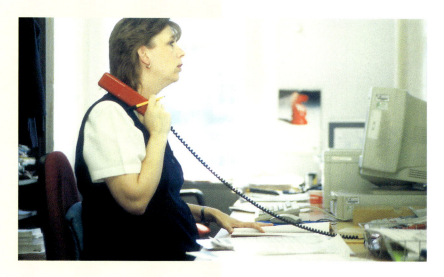

26 weeks by the 15th week before your baby is due you can also take a further 26 weeks Additional Maternity Leave (AML). AML is unpaid leave and starts at the end of OML, giving women who qualify for it up to one year off.

You must notify your employer of your pregnancy and the date you intend to start maternity leave by the 15th week before your baby is due. Your midwife or GP will give you the MAT B1 form, the maternity certificate 'proving' you are pregnant, which you should also send to your employer. Your employer must reply within four weeks of notification, giving you information on your entitlement.

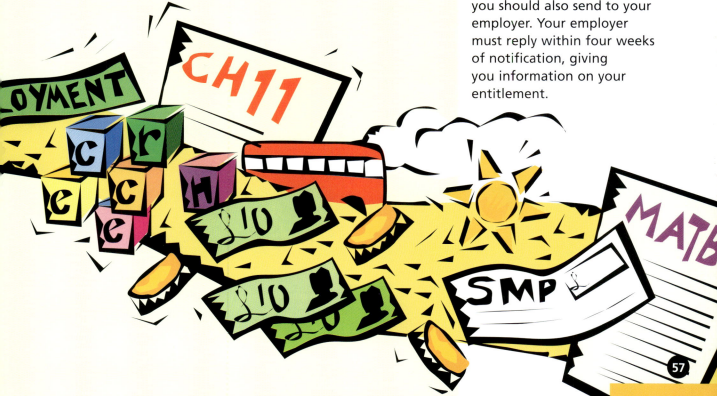

Your job is protected. It is illegal for your employer to dismiss you or make you redundant for any reason connected with your pregnancy, the birth, or your maternity leave. This applies no matter how many hours you work, and no matter how long you have worked for the same employer.

Some jobs and some workplaces may have agreed maternity rights that are better and more flexible than the ones laid down in law. You should always check with your contract of employment, your personnel department, or your trade union representative, to make sure of what you are entitled to.

Benefits and payments

Working out the money that's due to you during and after pregnancy is quite complicated.

Statutory Maternity Pay (SMP)

Statutory Maternity Pay (SMP) will be paid for 26 weeks. SMP will be paid at 90 per cent of your average earnings for 6 weeks and £100 per week (or 90 per cent of average weekly earnings if this is less) for 20 weeks. To qualify for SMP you will need to have worked for your employer for 26 weeks by the 15th week before your baby is due and earn over the National Insurance Lower Earnings Limit.

For up-to-date figures check with your employer, your union or your Citizens' Advice Bureau.

Maternity Allowance

If you do not qualify for SMP, for example because your earnings are too low, you can claim Maternity Allowance from the Benefits Agency. Maternity Allowance will be paid at the flat rate of £100 per week (or 90 per cent of average weekly earnings if this is less) for 26 weeks. To claim, you will need form MA1 from the Benefits Agency.

Parental Leave

There is already a right for both parents to take up to 13 weeks unpaid parental leave per parent per child. You must have worked for your employer for one year by the date you wish to take it. Parents can take parental leave after maternity or paternity leave providing they give 21 days notice.

When to leave, when to return?

These decisions are up to you. You can work right up to the day your baby is born if you wish, and you will still be entitled to the same amount of leave from your job — it just means it will all be taken after the birth instead of before.

Paternity Leave

Two weeks paid paternity leave is now in place for fathers of babies due on or after 6 April 2003. Statutory Paternity Pay (SPP) will be paid at a flat rate of £100 per week (or 90 per cent of average weekly earnings if this is less) for two weeks. Paternity leave can be taken from the date of birth or up to eight weeks from the birth. To qualify for SPP, your partner will need to have worked for his employer for 26 weeks by the 15th week before the baby is due and earn more than the Lower Earnings Limit. He must also give his employer notice of the date he wants to start paternity leave by the 15th week before the baby is due.

Child Benefit and One Parent Benefit

These benefits are payable from the date the baby is born. They come from the Benefits Agency. There is a form for Child Benefit on the back of their leaflet *Babies and Benefits*. You need form CH11 if you want to claim One Parent Benefit. Send the completed forms with your baby's birth certificate in the pre-paid envelope.

Sure Start Parents Payment

This is a lump sum grant for expectant mothers on Income Support, means-tested JobSeeker's Allowance, Family Credit or Disability Working Allowance. To qualify, parents are required to submit a certificate signed by an approved health professional confirming that advice has been sought on the needs of the new baby.

Your local Benefits Agency office can help you with more information. Also, see Further help at the back of this book.

WORKING AFTER YOUR BABY IS BORN

It's not easy being a working parent, no matter what age your child is when you decide to start work outside the home, or return to work. Finding high-quality childcare is important, of course, and if you plan on returning after a few months, you may want to look at your options while you are still pregnant.

- Anyone offering daycare to babies and young children should be registered with your local authority, including workplace nurseries or crèches. This ensures safety checks have been made, and that there is a correct ratio of staff to children. You can get a list of registered minders, nurseries and crèches in your area. Ask other parents about their experiences, and visit the minder or the nursery, with or without your child, as many times as you need to feel confident.

- When the day comes to leave your child, you are bound to have anxieties. It will help if you get your child used to the new carer or carers before you have to leave. But it can be an emotional time, and many parents feel pressures at being split from their work and from their need to be with their child.

- For information on continuing to breastfeed after your return to work, see page 97. A booklet entitled *Breastfeeding and Returning to Work* is available from your local health promotion department.

Twins

WILL PREGNANCY AND BIRTH BE DIFFERENT?

Twins (and more) are formed either by the egg splitting shortly after fertilisation (identical twins), or by two or more eggs being fertilised by two or more sperm (non-identical or fraternal twins). Non-identical twins are slightly more likely to happen after a course of fertility treatment which stimulates ovulation, and which means more than one egg may be released. They can also happen when more than one fertilised egg is put into the uterus after in-vitro fertilisation (test-tube pregnancy).

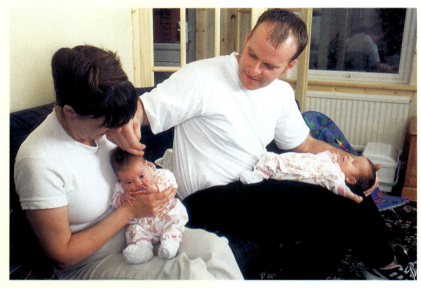

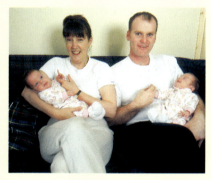

Twins may show up on the screen during an ultrasound scan. They may be suspected because your uterus is larger than expected at this stage of pregnancy.

The main concern of a multiple pregnancy, even if you are healthy and have no major problems, is that you may get double helpings of the minor discomforts of pregnancy. That means (for example) more backache, fatigue, heartburn and nausea, constipation and piles. The increased weight gain, and the excess of pregnancy hormones, contribute to this. Try to rest, especially later on in pregnancy. A healthy diet is particularly important.

Extra care

If you are expecting twins, or more, you will receive more attention during pregnancy.

The reasons for this extra care include:

- greater chance of high blood pressure, which needs careful observation, and possible treatment
- twins or more are likely to be born before 40 weeks — 37 or 38 weeks is average for twins, but 25 per cent of twin pregnancies end before 36 weeks

- birth problems are more common, and Caesarean section may be necessary to speed up delivery, or to deliver the second twin quickly. Less space in the uterus means one or both twins may be in a difficult, or impossible, position for a vaginal birth.

Triplet pregnancy is even more likely than twins to end in a pre-term, and/or operative delivery. Caesarean section is considered virtually inevitable for quads or quints, to speed up and control the delivery. Even so, while multiple pregnancy is hard work, and a multiple labour and delivery may be more of a challenge to everyone, especially you, the majority of twin and triplet births are as joyous and rewarding as any other, and many pregnancies and births are perfectly straightforward.

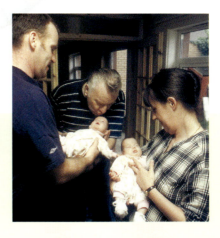

Q. **Is it possible to breastfeed twins?**

A. **Yes. Your body is capable of making as much milk as your babies need. Twins double the demand on the breast milk production, and therefore they double the supply. It is equally possible to breastfeed triplets (and more!).**

The practicalities, however, of feeding more than one baby are something of a challenge. The babies may be small and they may tire easily, so you may have to work quite hard at first in getting them interested in feeding. You may need skilled help to teach them to latch on well (see page 91). You'll need time to decide which is the best way of feeding — two together or separately. Even when you think you have got it sorted out, you may find you have to change to suit your babies' changing needs.

Twins tend to differ in their feeding habits, just as any other two babies might, and keeping them both happy may be hard in the early weeks. You need to feel confident, and to have encouragement from the people around you. You also need help with any other jobs in the house. In time, feeding becomes less intensive — and many women find it easier than making up bottles of formula milk.

Twins in the uterus — how do they lie?

The best presentation of twins is both head-down — 'cephalic' or 'vertex' — and is the most common. However, pressure of space in the uterus means it's also not uncommon for one or both babies to be breech (feet or bottom down). Transverse lie (baby across the uterus) is also a possibility, and if this is the case with the first presenting twin, a Caesarean section is inevitable. If the second twin is lying across, there may be an attempt to turn the second twin, after the first twin has been born vaginally.

MULTIPLE BIRTHS — THE STATISTICS

The birth of more than one baby is always known as a multiple birth, whether there are two, three or more. One baby at a time is known as a singleton.

- 1 pregnancy in every 80 is a twin pregnancy.

- 1 pregnancy in 8000 is triplets.

- 1 pregnancy in 800,000 is quads.

Multiple pregnancy tends to run in families, down the female line. The tendency to release more than one egg at ovulation seems to be inherited. The twins which 'run in families' are non-identical, because of this.

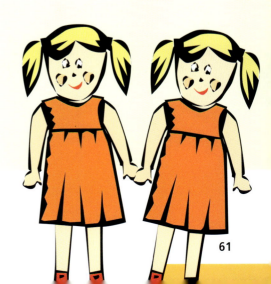

In touch with your baby

YOUR BABY'S 'EXPERIENCES'

It's known that unborn babies have some awareness of their surroundings, and may be able to respond to them.

Over the years, researchers have tried to study the responses of the unborn baby. It is possible to study some physical reactions to certain happenings.

A memory of the uterus?

Parents and unborn babies have been studied together and followed up after the birth. This work points to the possibility that babies have some sort of memory of their life in the womb.

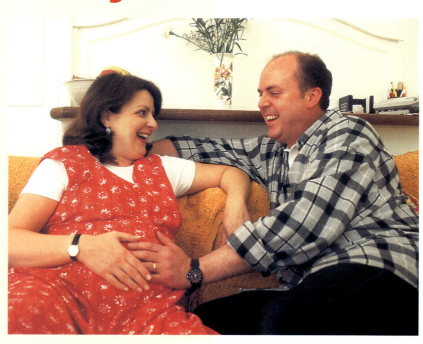

In one study, some pregnant mothers had the habit of relaxing with a cup of tea and a well-known soap opera on the television, each afternoon in late pregnancy. After they were born, their babies were found to relax whenever the researchers played them the soap's signature tune.

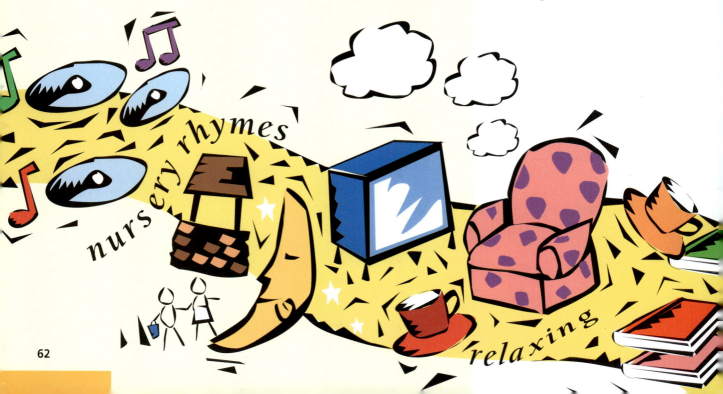

nursery rhymes

relaxing

Your baby can dream — maybe

The nerve pathways of the brain are as developed in a baby of just 28 weeks gestation as they are in a baby at term. From week 32, tests can detect REM (rapid eye movement) sleep in a baby. In adults, REM sleep means the person is dreaming. Researchers think that the unborn baby may be reliving, by this dreaming, some of the experiences of moving, of hearing, of seeing and feeling, in preparation for life outside the womb.

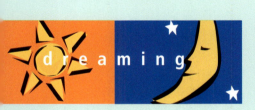

What you can do

● Play music regularly to your baby — perhaps set aside a time, say 10 minutes a few times a week, for this. The research shows that unborn babies are more restful, as if listening, when simple melodies are played.

● You and your partner can talk to your baby, while lying down and relaxing. Your baby can hear your voice, and can get to know it better when it's not competing with other noises. It doesn't matter what you say, but use a calm, regular tone of voice. Try reciting nursery rhymes if you don't know what to say.

● The fetus is sensitive to touch from very early on in the pregnancy. In the second half of pregnancy, you can feel clear movements. You can touch and massage your abdomen — gently and regularly. You can use a vegetable oil such as almond oil, or a light moisturising cream, to make it more pleasant for you. Your partner can share in the massage.

'I used to talk to our baby when I was on my own. It just felt natural to me, to have a little chat from time to time. I would tell him how much we were looking forward to him coming to be with us, and what we'd do together. I found it was very relaxing, and calming, for me to do this.'

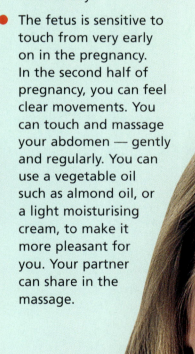

Antenatal classes

WHAT'S ON OFFER, HOW TO CHOOSE?

About half of all pregnant women attend some antenatal or preparation for parenthood classes. A typical class will form part of a course of six to eight, which you'd go to towards the end of your pregnancy. There are many variations. Some classes are open and 'rolling' — you can join at any time and leave at any time. Some classes are specially designed for different groups of mothers — teenage mothers, for example, or mothers from the same ethnic background.

Antenatal classes cover a wide range of topics, but in most you can expect to hear about:

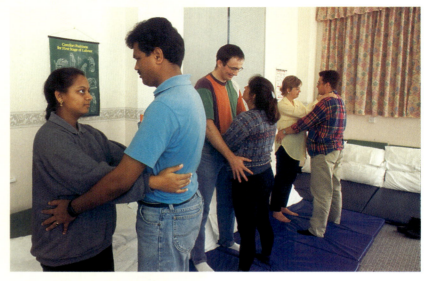

- health in pregnancy, with advice on diet and coping with minor discomforts

- what to expect in later pregnancy, and in labour and birth
- pain relief options
- coping with labour and birth using self-help techniques such as relaxation and breathing
- possible problems with labour and birth
- Caesarean section, forceps, ventouse delivery
- exercises for pregnancy, birth and afterwards
- baby feeding

- caring for your baby in the early days and weeks
- birth plans.

Most clinics, hospitals and health centres have antenatal classes. They are free, and are usually run by midwives and/or health visitors. Other non-NHS classes may charge a fee. They're run by specially trained antenatal teachers, who may also be, but usually are not, health professionals. They are almost always mothers themselves. NHS classes are usually held in a room in the clinic itself — other classes may be in the teacher's own home.

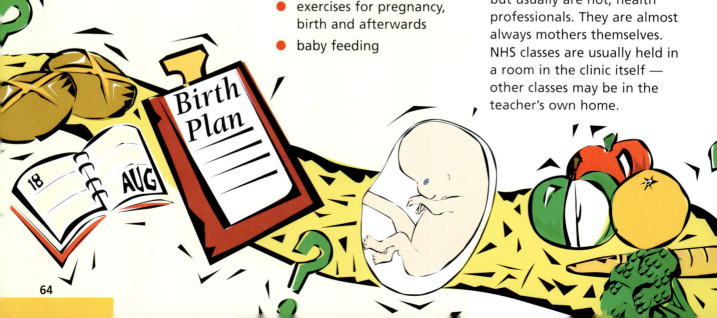

Q. How do I find out what's available to me locally?

A. Your midwife or health visitor is a good source of information. Any health professional can find out where the local clinic or hospital classes are, and their times and dates. For information about National Childbirth Trust classes, and classes run by members of the Scottish Birth Teachers Association, or others, see the addresses at the back of this book, or try your local telephone book.

Q. What about payment for non-NHS classes?

A. Fees for non-NHS classes vary, but on the whole, teachers don't like to feel that women might be put off from coming because they can't afford the fees. There are often subsidised class fees, or paying by easy instalments. In some cases, fees may not be charged at all. Just ask at the time of booking.

A good antenatal class will be much more than someone standing at the front talking to you. It will:

- encourage you to ask about, and discuss, things that are important to you
- explain everything in a way you understand
- help you face labour, birth and early parenthood with confidence.

It will offer support and encouragement in a warm, friendly atmosphere so you can make new friends and feel the rest of the class is supporting you, too.

Choosing the right class is easier if you ask around first. The midwife will know about classes, and which ones have good reports. If you know mothers who have given birth recently, ask them if they went to any good classes. You can go to more than one set of classes, if you wish.

Your partner at antenatal classes

Some antenatal classes are run for couples and while they may be happy to have mothers only along, too, you may feel a little uncomfortable if you are the only one on your own. Consider taking a friend along instead.

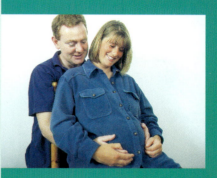

Some antenatal courses have a couples session or 'men only' sessions.

It's up to you and your partner, if you have one, to decide what's right for you. Some partners are quite adamant they don't want to go to any of the classes, and some mothers-to-be prefer to be on their own. Sharing in an antenatal class is a good way for partners to meet others who may have similar concerns, and it gives them a chance to ask questions, too. Partners can find out how to support you at the birth, and during breastfeeding. You can practise massage and relaxation techniques, and make new friends as a couple.

If your partner is a woman, your relationship can be kept confidential, or not, just as you prefer. Female friends and relatives often accompany women to classes.

Preparing for your baby

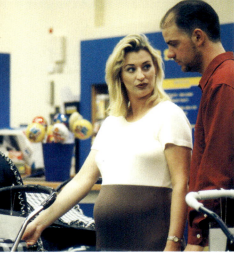

WHAT YOU WILL NEED

You don't have to buy everything your baby needs in one go. Lots of baby equipment isn't needed until much later. Babies need clothes, nappies, somewhere warm and clean to sleep, something to 'ride' in like a baby carrier, pram or pushchair (with a lie-back position), bedding, a car safety seat if you use a car — and that's it for the first few months.

Bottle-fed babies need bottles and sterilising equipment (see pages 99–101).

Optional extras in the very early weeks

- Baby carrier or sling.

- Baby bath — useful but not essential. Your baby can use the big bath, or even a clean washing-up bowl in the first week or two.

- Crib/Moses basket — pretty and easier to move than the 'big' cot, but soon outgrown.

- Cuddly toys — attractive in the baby's room, but of no interest to your baby for the first months.

- Changing mat or table — any clean, covered flat surface, including the floor, or your lap, can be used for your baby's nappy changes (if you have had a Caesarean section, you'll need a raised surface, such as a mat on top of a changing unit or dressing table).

- Breast pump — you won't need this straight away, and in any case, hand expressing of breast milk, without using a pump, is a useful skill to learn (see page 98).

For some suggestions about the clothing your baby will need, see page 113.

You can save money if you:

- buy second hand where possible. Check equipment for stability and safety (see also page 114)

- use hand-me-downs — good baby clothing can be used for several babies

- don't buy newborn-sized baby clothes. The next size up may look big, but your baby doesn't care. (Small or pre-term babies will need some newborn clothing, though.)

- cut down old bed sheets and hem them for cot and pram bedding

- borrow equipment which you'll need for no more than a few weeks or months, or share the cost with a friend or relative whose baby is due some months before or after yours.

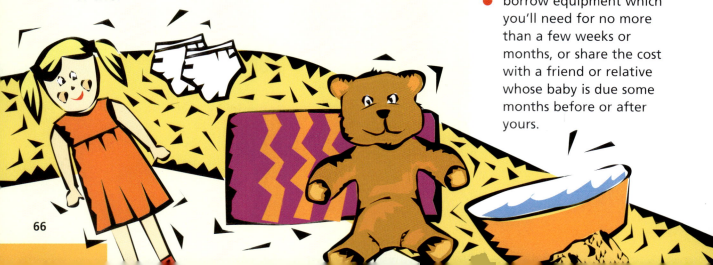

Pre-term labour

WHEN YOUR BABY ARRIVES EARLY

Pre-term labour is generally defined as labour beginning before the 37th week of pregnancy. Over the last few years, babies born early have had a greater chance of surviving and developing without any long-term problems. The outlook for a pre-term baby is affected by:

- the number of weeks you are pregnant (the later, the better)

- the baby's size. Bigger babies usually have a better chance of survival, as long as they are healthy in other ways

- whether the baby has any birth abnormality

- the availability of specialist care.

It is very rare for any baby to survive more than a short time if born before 23 weeks. At 24 weeks, just under half of all babies survive. A baby born at 25 weeks has a slightly higher than 50 per cent chance of survival. At 26 weeks, 75 per cent, and at 28 weeks, 85 per cent of babies survive. By the time the pregnancy has reached the 35th week, the baby is likely to be fine, but may have to spend some time in special care. Some pre-term babies survive but have a permanent or long-term disability or health problem.

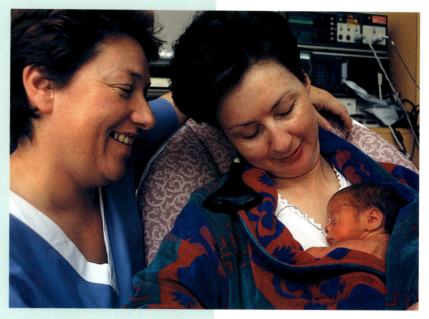

Why are some babies born early?

It's not always known why some women go into labour early. There are several possible reasons:

- infection in the mother

- conditions such as pre-eclampsia

- more than one baby. Most twins and triplets are born before 38 weeks, and many sooner than this. The uterus starts to contract when it is over-stretched

- weakness in the cervix.

If your labour starts early, you will either experience rupture of the membranes (your waters will 'break'), or you will start to feel contractions. If you suspect you are in labour, or if you are bleeding, call the hospital straight away.

It may be possible to slow down or even stop your labour. Drugs that stop you contracting may give your baby more time in the uterus. You may also be given treatment to prevent your baby being born with respiratory distress syndrome, a condition which seriously affects breathing.

Occasionally, a mother might be advised she needs to have her labour induced because she has a condition that threatens her health, or her baby's health. Or, her baby might be thought to have a better chance of health or survival outside the uterus (see page 75 for more information on induction).

For information about your baby in special care, see page 29.

When pregnancy goes wrong

LOSING YOUR BABY BEFORE BIRTH

As many as one in four pregnancies miscarry, though the usual figure given is about one in six confirmed pregnancies. A miscarriage is defined as the loss of the fetus before 24 weeks. About one baby in every 200 is stillborn (dies in the uterus after 24 weeks).

Some pregnancies end after termination for abnormality.

Miscarriage

The medical term for a miscarriage is a 'spontaneous abortion'. Most miscarriages happen in the first three months, and most miscarriages have no clear cause. We know that early miscarriages — before 12 weeks of pregnancy — are usually the result of a 'blighted ovum' when the pregnancy does not develop correctly, for no apparent reason.

Sometimes, the pregnancy has ended, but the embryo remains in the uterus. This is called a missed abortion. In time it would be expelled without any intervention, although a short minor operation called an 'evacuation of uterus' is often offered. This would be done under an anaesthetic.

Occasionally, miscarriages are caused by a condition called cervical incompetence. This means that the cervix doesn't stay closed. It starts to dilate, while the uterus contracts. The baby is lost before about the 20th week.

Ectopic pregnancy

The pregnancy has developed outside the uterus, usually in the fallopian tube (see pages 17 and 35).

Hydatidiform mole

This is not a true pregnancy, but a collection of fluid-filled sacs growing from the tissue that would have become the placenta. The mole is removed by an operation, or by inducing the uterus to expel it.

Stillbirth

Some babies die in the uterus, or at birth, but this is very uncommon. This could be because of a serious abnormality. Or the placenta may have stopped functioning well, and the baby lacks oxygen as a result. Often, it's just not known why the baby dies.

Saying goodbye to your baby

With later miscarriage, and stillbirth, you will give birth to your baby, after a labour and delivery. Many parents find it helpful to hold their baby, when possible. This acknowledges the depth of grief at the loss of a real little person, who was wanted and who would have been welcomed with love. You can dress or wrap your baby and care for her tenderly. A midwife or doctor can take a picture for you. You may not want to hold your baby straight away, but a sensitive midwife will ask you once or twice if you want to — so many parents later treasure the memory that she will want to make sure you have the chance to say yes.

Ask the hospital what arrangements can be made for a funeral, or you can arrange your own. The hospital chaplain can be a good source of support and information, whether or not you are religious.

Your midwife or doctor may ask your permission to carry out a post-mortem examination on your baby. This may help give information about why your baby died. A post-mortem is always done sensitively, and you will hardly notice any effects of it.

Q. I have had two early miscarriages, and I have been told just to try again. How can I make sure I don't lose another baby, if I get pregnant again?

A. The usual medical definition of 'recurrent miscarriage' is when three or more miscarriages have happened in succession. Having two miscarriages is very distressing for you, but it's probably nothing to do with any underlying condition. You have a very high chance of carrying your next pregnancy to term. However, you will need emotional support, as the next pregnancy is likely to be an anxious time for you.

Emotional support after pregnancy loss

Other women who have lost babies may be a great support for you. Just knowing you are not alone can mean a great deal. With other people who understand, you don't have to pretend to be brave. See **Further help** at the back of this book for the addresses and phone numbers of groups who can help.

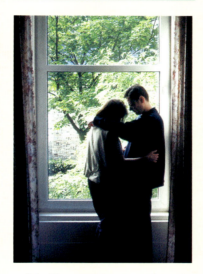

Your midwife, and your GP, can offer you support, and should be able to go through your notes with you, to help you understand, if it's possible, why you lost your baby, and reassure you that you are in no way to blame. After a late miscarriage or a stillbirth, you will need midwifery care, to make sure your body is recovering from the pregnancy.

People may tend to think about the mother most after a miscarriage or a stillbirth, but partners need support, too. Your partner may also be the main link between you and the health professionals, which can be very stressful.

'I felt I was the only one to have lost a baby — I'd hardly heard the word "stillbirth" before in my life. Then, when I met people, they didn't seem to know what to say to me. I could see people crossing the road rather than talk to me. I felt so alone. I suppose they were too embarrassed — but it felt like they just didn't care. Or they cared more about their own embarrassment than my pain.'

BECOMING PREGNANT AGAIN

If you have recently lost a baby, you may not want to think about becoming pregnant again for a while, if ever; or you may yearn to fill the empty space in your arms, and your life, with another baby. People's feelings differ. There's no 'right' or 'normal' way to feel.

There's no 'right' time to become pregnant again, either. Medically, about three to six months is the time needed to allow your body to recover and to establish a menstrual cycle. But emotionally, this may be too soon for you. Only you know what's right — some couples want to leave space to allow for grieving. It can be hard to look forward to a new birth when you are still so sad about the baby you lost.

WILL IT HAPPEN AGAIN?

Most causes of stillbirths, neonatal deaths and miscarriages are unlikely to recur. But there are a few causes which could recur, and you will be offered information on what to expect.

Sometimes, pre-conception care or genetic counselling can help next time, especially if you are concerned that either you or your partner may have a health problem or an inherited condition that could affect pregnancy. Your doctor can refer you to a specialist in this sort of care.

Labour

WHAT TO LOOK OUT FOR

Your labour and birth are unique and women's experiences vary — all normal, but none predictable. The beginning of labour is often not clear-cut, and sometimes it can start without you being fully aware of it. The first signs of labour can happen within a few hours of each other, or they could be spread out over a longer period of time. The obvious signs are:

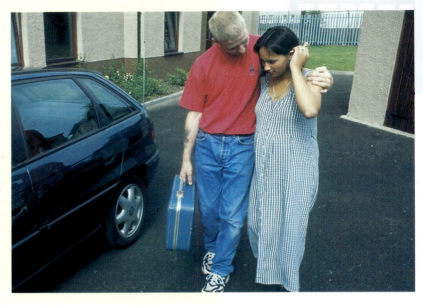

- **the 'show':** this is the release of the mucus plug, or operculum, which seals the opening of the cervix. In some women it comes out of the vagina as a single blob of pinkish jelly; in others it is a series of smaller pieces, and in others it can be reddish brown and blood-tinged. It is a sign that the cervix is beginning to stretch and soften a little, in preparation for labour. It may not mean you are actually in labour. It can be several days between the show and the start of labour proper, or just an hour or so, or anything in between

- **'breaking of the waters':** the membranes, or amniotic sac, is the bag of fluid surrounding the baby inside the uterus. When the membranes break, or rupture, the fluid escapes. It can happen as a sudden gush of liquid down your legs. More usually, though, it will start to trickle. Telephone your doctor, midwife or the hospital if your waters break. There may be a risk of infection to the baby if the membranes rupture

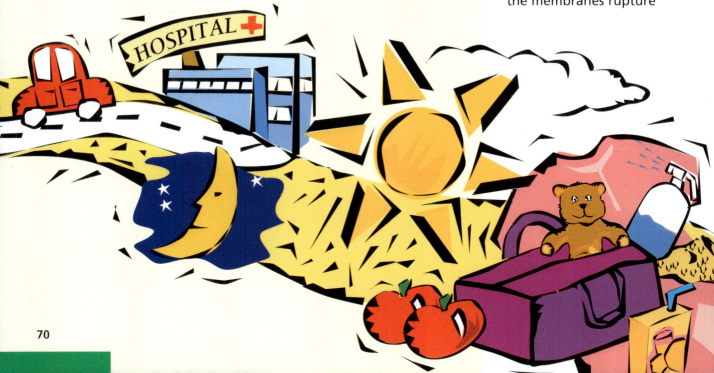

and labour doesn't start within a day or so. If the baby's head is not yet engaged, or if your baby is breech, a rush of waters may bring the cord with it. The cord could then become compressed, which would be risky for your baby's oxygen supply

- **contractions:** these are the only sure signs of labour if they gradually come closer together and last longer than 40 seconds. You should feel them getting stronger, longer and more rhythmical, too.

If you're not sure what to do, contact the maternity unit where you plan to give birth, or your community midwife. Describe your symptoms, and you will be advised on whether you need to do anything other than wait and see what happens over the next few hours. You may have a visit from a midwife, whether or not you plan a home birth, who can examine you if necessary, and help you decide where the best place is for you.

WHAT IS A CONTRACTION?

The uterus is a network of muscle fibres, and contractions happen when the fibres shorten. They do this to pull up the cervix and to press down at the top of the uterus. The muscles relax as the contraction dies away. With each contraction the muscles stay shorter than they were. This leaves the cervix slightly more open and pushes the baby a little further down.

Contractions usually feel like a tightening sensation across your tummy and possibly into your back and thighs. They usually begin gently, build up to a peak and then trail off. They may remind you of period pains (which are also contractions of the uterus), or feel much more painful. Women have different experiences with contractions, as the intensity can vary a lot.

Sometimes women can start to have contractions only for them to fade away. This can be deceptive, and many women think they are in labour. They go to hospital, only to find everything stops. If this happens to you, you may be examined, and you may be disappointed that you are not very far on in your labour; maybe your cervix doesn't show that the contractions have had any effect at all.

In this situation, you may be asked if you'd prefer to go home. This is sensible, unless you live a long way from the hospital. Don't feel embarrassed. This sort of false alarm happens all the time.

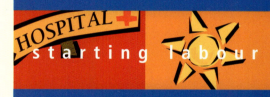

HOSPITAL

starting labour

SEX AND LABOUR

There is a widespread idea that sexual activity can start labour, when the baby is ready to be born. There may be some basis to this. Semen has natural prostaglandins (hormones) in it, and may stimulate the cervix to 'ripen' a little more. Sexual stimulation in the woman releases hormones — oxytocins — which are released in labour, too. There's no evidence that any sexual activity starts labour too soon. If labour was about to begin anyway, then this helps it a little.

The first stage

WHAT'S HAPPENING?

Labour is usually divided into three stages. The first stage is usually the longest, but anything between an hour and 20 hours or longer is normal.

At the start of the first stage, you may be getting one contraction of 40 or 50 seconds every 10 minutes. At the end, each contraction will usually last longer than a minute, and there will be a gap of no more than a minute between each one. This pattern may vary, though.

At the beginning, labour often progresses quite slowly. When you are five to six centimetres dilated, contractions are longer and stronger and labour progresses more quickly. This is called 'established' labour.

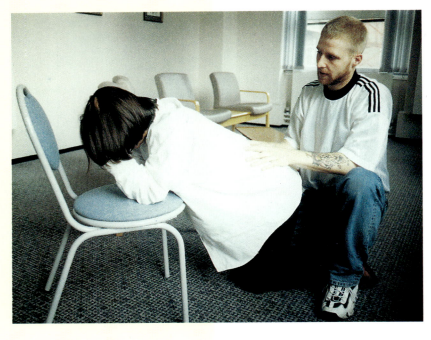

Contractions help to open the cervix. When open, contractions help the uterus to push the baby out. By the end of the first stage, the cervix is fully open, and is completely taken up by the uterus.

At 10 centimetres dilated your cervix is fully dilated, and you are ready for the birth.

Labour probably begins as a result of hormonal impulses, triggered by the baby — we don't know for sure. When the baby's adrenal gland is mature, the baby secretes cortisone. This alters the levels of oestrogen and progesterone in the mother, and as a result she starts to produce hormone-like chemicals called prostaglandins. These stimulate the uterus to start contracting.

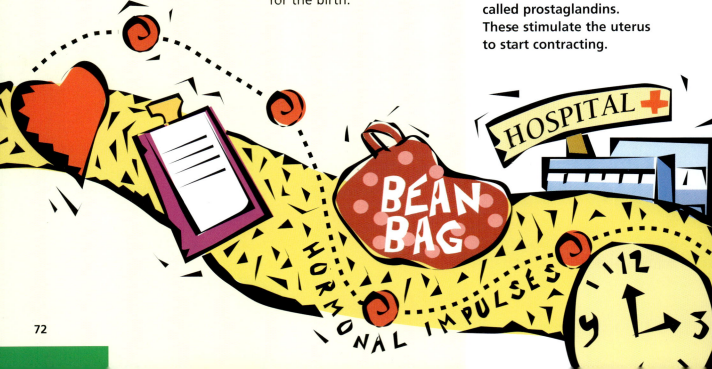

COPING WITH LABOUR

Labour is like a journey up a high mountain or some other challenge you've faced. Sometimes, you may be able to view the peak. At other times it is hidden, and you may forget the aim of the whole exercise. But each step takes you closer to the peak.

Contractions are steps on that journey. Think of each contraction as a means to an end ... bringing you closer to the birth of your baby. Contractions are usually painful, but between contractions you probably won't feel much pain at all.

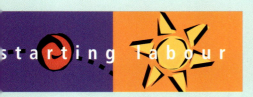

As you feel a contraction coming ...

- relax. Think especially about your shoulders, your face, your hands. Make sure they are 'unclenched'

Q. **Can I eat in labour?**

A. **You will have to ask your midwife about the policy in your unit.**

The traditional 'rule' on food in labour was that women should not eat anything, just in case they needed a general anaesthetic. In some units, this rule is now relaxed.

- start to concentrate on your breathing, keeping it slow and relaxed. Focus on breathing out

- as the contraction gets stronger, think more carefully about the way you breathe and try to stay relaxed

- sway and rock your pelvis; make any noises you find helpful

- don't resist the contraction — it increases in intensity, it reaches its height, it starts to fade ...

- ... as it goes, blow it away. It's gone. That contraction will never appear again, and it's one less on your journey.

Most women cope best with labour if they are not restricted in their movements. You may find different positions — kneeling, leaning forwards on a beanbag or your partner's lap, on all fours and anything else that helps — work best for you at different times. Listen to your body, experiment with different movements, do what's most helpful for you.

MONITORING YOUR BABY

Measuring the baby's heart rate is a way of assessing your baby's health and strength throughout labour and birth.

Different ways of monitoring

- **A Pinard stethoscope** is a type of ear-trumpet, placed against your abdomen to listen to the baby's heart. It is used from time to time during labour.

- **A 'doppler'** is a smaller, portable machine using ultrasound for monitoring at intervals. A small transmitter-receiver is placed on your abdomen to pick up the heartbeat.

- **Electronic fetal monitoring (EFM)** uses ultrasound waves to transmit your baby's heart rate to a machine via a 'transducer' held against your abdomen. Alternatively, a small electrode can be clipped on to your baby's scalp (or the bottom, in a breech baby) and this picks up and transmits the heartbeat. The heart rate usually appears in digital form on the screen, and a record is traced on graph paper and printed out.

- **Telemetry** uses the same sort of transducer or scalp electrode, but sends signals by radio waves to the receiver. You're not actually attached to the monitor by wires, so you are free to move around as long as you stay within its range.

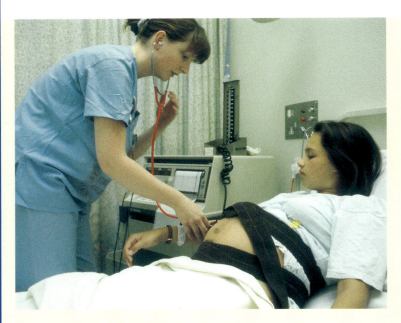

Electronic fetal monitoring

EFM provides continuous monitoring of the baby. In individual cases, this can be important — when the baby is at risk, or if it's known that there could be a problem.

Continuous EFM is not very useful in uncomplicated labour. Interpreting the monitor reading is a highly skilled job. Even very experienced obstetricians differ about what is a 'normal' reading, and what might give cause for concern. In many hospitals, doctors and midwives agree that continuous EFM is not needed for routine, normal labour, especially not in the first stage. Instead, mothers may be offered monitoring when first admitted to hospital, at intervals afterwards, and during the second stage.

EFM is necessary when an intervention such as induction, syntocinon or epidural is undertaken as these may cause stress to the baby.

If you and your carers expect everything to be normal, you may prefer to have the other forms of monitoring — intermittent monitoring with a doppler, or a Pinard stethoscope. You'll probably find your baby's heart is listened to every 15 or 20 minutes or so, and after most contractions in second stage.

OTHER CHECKS YOU WILL HAVE

Your condition and the baby's will be assessed when you are admitted to the labour ward, and at intervals throughout the first stage. These are the things which are regularly assessed:

- your blood pressure, your pulse and your temperature

- your urine, which helps the midwife to check your energy levels

- the length, strength and frequency of your contractions

- your cervix, during an internal or vaginal examination. Today, many midwives avoid vaginal examination as a routine. They do this only if they feel the information it gives will be useful.

WHAT IF CONTRACTIONS SLOW DOWN OR STOP?

Sometimes, labour seems to come to a stop. If you and your baby are well, there is no need for concern. Be patient, walk around, change your position, relax with some music ... your contractions will probably start up again in time. You may feel you want to eat something. This is your body's way of telling you that you need more 'fuel' to keep going.

If your labour is very slow, and perhaps because your baby is showing signs of distress, your doctor may advise speeding up your labour. This is called **augmentation** or **acceleration** of labour.

- Your contractions may be stimulated by artificial rupture of the membranes (ARM) if your waters are still unbroken.

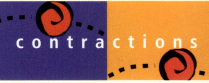

- You may be offered a hormone drip, which puts syntocinon directly into your bloodstream. The effect can be quite powerful — the contractions become much stronger than before and more frequent. You may not want this — most mothers cope better with a gradual build-up.

Unless it's essential that things speed up, you may prefer not to have any interventions.

An 'extra' stage of labour, sometimes known as 'transition' comes between first and second stage. Many women clearly experience it as different from other parts of their labour. You may feel the beginning of an urge to push. Alternatively, labour seems to stop.

Transition is a psychological state as well as a physical one. You might feel impatient, and tired, even angry, frustrated or irritable with your carers. This is a perfectly natural reaction and it also means that the birth of your baby is not far off.

YOUR POSITION

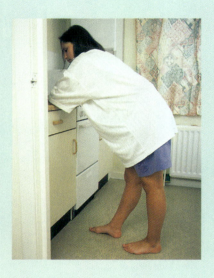

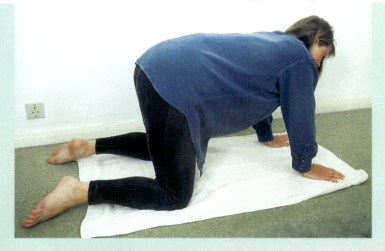

All-fours: you can rest by leaning forward between contractions.

On your side: you lie on your side (the 'lateral' position), with your upper leg raised. This is quite helpful if you are extremely tired.

Supported standing or squatting allows your pelvis to open wide, and your baby to be born with the help of the force of gravity. You will need support for your upper body to keep your balance. Your partner can support you by holding you from behind, under your arms, though it will need strength to take all your weight. Your knees must never be higher than your hips — this would put too much strain on your joints.

There's no right or wrong position. However, lying on your back is usually uncomfortable and closes your pelvis. When women are encouraged to do what feels best, they hardly ever adopt this position.

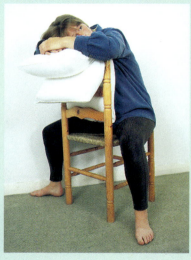

Sitting: astride a chair and leaning forward, resting on a cushion or pillow.

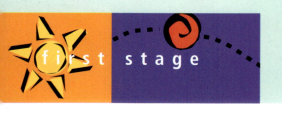

first stage

Sitting up in bed is an alternative to lying down but still puts some pressure on the pelvis. If you choose this position use plenty of pillows to support your back and shoulders. Your partner can easily hold you, supporting you behind the shoulders while sitting next to the bed.

The second stage

YOUR BABY IS ALMOST HERE

Second stage begins when the cervix is fully dilated, and ends with the birth of the baby.

You will probably feel a powerful need to push down. It's called 'bearing down'. You may feel when the time is right to push, or your midwife can guide you. You may want to push about three times in each contraction. If you want to hold your breath to bear down, don't hold it too long.

Some women don't feel the urge to bear down, and in some labours it isn't necessary — the baby is born without any effort. If you have an epidural, you may not feel the urge to push, or not as strongly. The midwife will

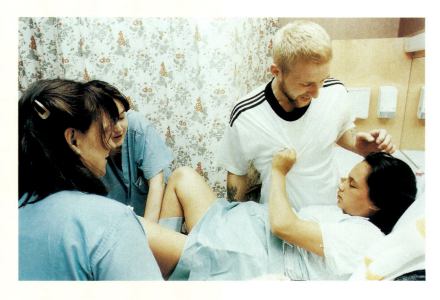

tell you when you should bear down.

As the head stretches the birth canal and the perineum (the skin between the birth canal and the anus), you may feel a powerful, burning sensation. It only lasts a short time. When the head can be seen completely at the vulva, it is said to be 'crowning'.

You can hold a mirror up if you want to, so you can see this moment.

You may feel your perineum stretching at this point. If there is a risk of tearing the perineum, your carers may ask you not to push now. You may be asked to pant, or to push more gently — to 'breathe the baby out' with lighter, gentler breaths.

With the next contraction or two, your baby's head comes out, and then your baby's body is born.

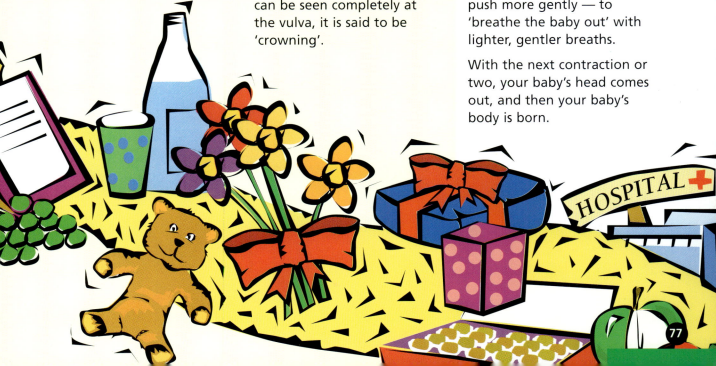

THE MOMENT OF BIRTH

During second stage, your baby's head turns, usually from facing to one side to facing towards your back.

As your baby's head comes out, the midwife may feel for the umbilical cord, to make sure it is not round the neck. You may be asked to relax or to pant at this point.

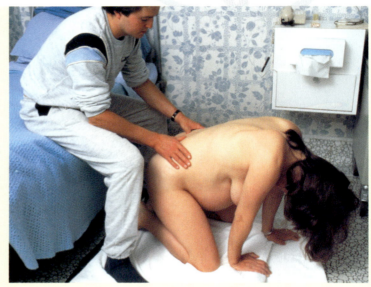

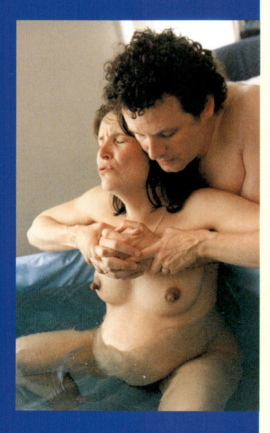

The shoulders turn so the body is sideways on, and the head, now fully born, faces towards your leg. Your baby then comes out easily and quickly.

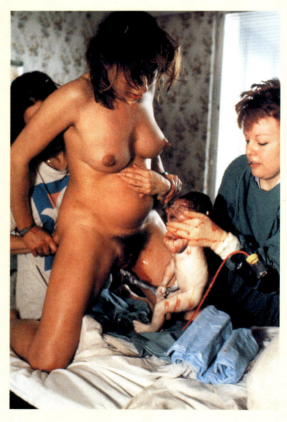

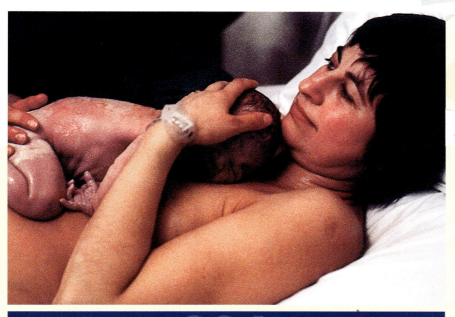

Your baby may have vernix on the skin — a creamy substance which helped to moisturise the skin in the uterus. There may be a few streaks of blood on the body (your blood, from your episiotomy or tear if you had one). The baby's head may look slightly misshapen, but this won't last long. It's called moulding — the soft bones of the skull have shaped themselves so that the baby's head can pass through the birth canal.

questions answered

Q. I know most fathers just take it for granted that they are going to be there during labour and birth. But I can't bear the idea. I know I'll be okay about the baby, and I'm looking forward to being a father. I just don't want to see it happen.

A. It's worth working out why you don't want to be there. Are you worried about being squeamish or even fainting? Or do you feel you won't want to look at the moment of birth, seeing the baby emerge? Or do you worry about what you're supposed to do, and whether you'll do it wrong? All these anxieties are common, and normal.

Talk over your feelings with your partner. If you decide to be there, you can always look away, and concentrate on your partner's face if watching the 'birth end' gets too much. You can leave the room if you need to.

During labour, you may not actually 'do' very much at times. That doesn't matter. Being there is more important. If you end up deciding you won't be there, your partner may need someone who can support her at the birth, and someone who can go to classes with her.

How long does second stage last?

With a first baby, the second stage can last between 10 minutes and a couple of hours or longer. Second or other babies may come after just a few pushes and one or two contractions.

ASSISTING BIRTH

In some situations, forceps or ventouse (vacuum) extraction are used to assist the baby's birth. It can happen when:

- the baby is short of oxygen — called fetal distress. It's diagnosed when the baby's heart rate slows in response to contractions, and doesn't speed up again as it should. A further sign is if the baby's bowels open and pass meconium (the contents of the baby's bowels). This will stain the amniotic fluid a green or brown colour. A small blood sample taken from the baby's scalp can be looked at and measured for oxygen

- the baby's exit is blocked or hampered — the position may be difficult, such as face-up (occipito-posterior), or the mother's pelvis may not be able to open wide enough, sometimes due to her position

- contractions have weakened

- the baby is pre-term, which means the head needs more protection

- the baby is breech, which may mean the head needs protection

- the mother is too tired to push

- the mother has a condition such as a heart disorder, and should not push for too long.

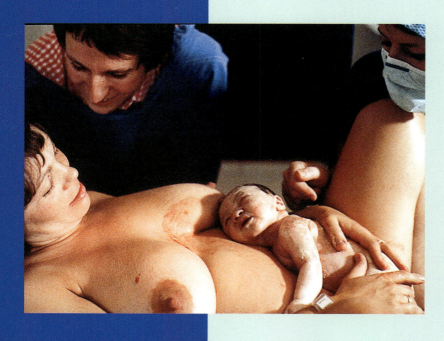

If you need help with forceps or ventouse

You will probably be asked to lie down on your back, and your legs will be raised, with the ankles supported in stirrups.

You will be given an anaesthetic, most likely an epidural or a spinal, or a local anaesthetic called a pudendal block, though a general anaesthetic is very occasionally used. Your bladder may be emptied with a catheter. You will probably need an episiotomy to allow room for the instrument to be inserted.

Forceps are made of two separate halves which lock on to one another. They have handles at one end, and two scoop-like blades at the other. The forceps are inserted into the vagina, one blade at a time. Each blade fits snugly over the sides of the baby's head, cupping it. The handles then lock, forming a protective cage round the head. The forceps turn the baby (if necessary).

Then, as you feel each contraction coming you push, just as you were doing, and the doctor coordinates the pulling.

Q. **Will I need stitches after the birth?**

A. **Sometimes the perineum tears while stretching over the baby's head. Or the midwife may ask if she can cut the perineum because you are about to tear badly, or the baby needs to be born quickly. This cut is known as an 'episiotomy'. There is some difference of opinion among midwives as to how often one should be done, although most would agree that it should only be used as an emergency procedure.**

A small tear usually heals itself. Larger ones, and episiotomies, may need stitching. You will be given a local anaesthetic while this is done. The stitches should dissolve themselves — you don't usually need to have them taken out. Until this happens, it's normal to have a few days of discomfort when you sit down. Tell the midwife if you have more pain than this. Sometimes taking out a stitch or two can help.

Ventouse extraction can turn and deliver the baby. It has a tube with a cup on it at one end. The tube leads to a small vacuum pump. The cup is attached to the baby's head by suction. The mother pushes with each contraction and the doctor pulls.

Your baby may show bruising on each side of the head where the forceps have been. Ventouse extraction can cause swelling (sometimes called a 'chignon') on the head. None of this is permanent, and it will disappear over the next few days.

The third stage

THE FIRST MOMENTS AFTER THE BIRTH

The third stage of labour is the delivery of the placenta and the membranes after your baby's birth. For most women, the third stage passes uneventfully. You might hardly be aware of it happening. In most hospitals the third stage is **'actively managed'**. This means some actions are routinely taken to speed up this stage of labour.

- First, you may have an injection to cause the uterus to contract. It is given when your baby is being born, usually when the first shoulder is coming out. The injection goes into your thigh or your buttock. The midwife will ask you for your consent before she does it.

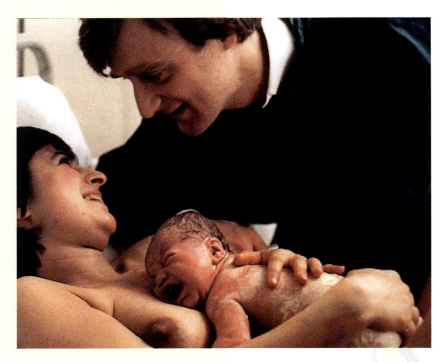

- The second action happens when your baby is born. The umbilical cord is clamped and cut. It's usual to make sure that the baby is breathing well, and is no longer dependent on the placenta for oxygen. **If you have not had an injection** the cord may

be cut now, or left until it stops pulsating or until after the delivery of the placenta.

- As the injection now takes effect, it stimulates the uterus into contracting very strongly, becoming smaller, harder and tighter. This causes the placenta to peel off the inner wall of the uterus. The contraction may make you want to push again, and you may

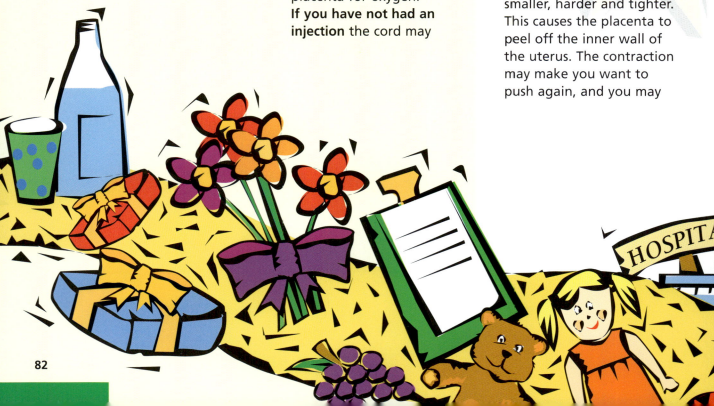

be able to push the placenta out. More usually, the doctor or midwife helps the delivery of the placenta. They put one hand on your abdomen to protect the uterus, while keeping the cord taut with the other hand. This is called 'cord traction'.

● The placenta comes away and the blood vessels which were 'holding on' to the placenta close off as the muscle in your uterus contracts. This prevents bleeding (though it's normal to bleed a little). You may feel the placenta slide down and out between your legs, followed by the membranes.

Occasionally, the placenta does not come away from the uterus. When this happens, the mother needs a small operation to remove it, which is always done under anaesthetic.

Another possible complication of the third stage is bleeding, called 'postpartum haemorrhage' or PPH. A haemorrhage needs to be treated immediately.

An unaided, or natural (also called a 'physiological') third stage happens without an injection or cord traction and can take some time. The action of feeding your baby at the breast or simply having the baby there in skin to skin contact with you, stimulates the release of the hormone oxytocin. This helps your uterus to contact and to push out the placenta and the membranes. The cord is cut when it stops pulsating, and often after the placenta is delivered.

You may want to discuss the third stage and whether it is actively managed or not when making your birth plan. If you have any problems during the first or second stage of this labour, or had any during or after a previous delivery, then a natural third stage may not be a safe option. Discuss this with your midwife.

Your baby's Apgar score: soon after the birth your midwife assesses your baby's well-being with the Apgar score. It's done by observation, usually at one minute and five minutes after the birth. Some units do a two-minute assessment only. Your baby's breathing, colour, muscle tone, response to stimulation and heart rate are checked, and given a mark of 0,1, or 2 for these aspects of the baby's appearance and health.

Greeting your baby

If everything is okay with you and with your baby, you can hold your baby straight away after the birth.

Cuddle your baby close to you, without any wrapping or clothing between you (skin to skin). The midwife will gently dry the baby and may place a cover over both you for warmth. Now isn't the time for wrapping your baby up. Instead, hold him close, and marvel in every inch of him! He is likely to want to be close to your breast, and you can offer him his first breastfeed (see over the page).

This close contact between you has been shown to help breastfeeding get off to a good start. It also helps your baby to stay warm, he hears your heartbeat as he would in the womb, his blood circulation to his hands and feet will be better than if he was in a cot, and he is less likely to cry. Just enjoy this special time, and don't let yourself feel there is any rush. Talk to your baby, and gaze at him, and relish these loving moments — you'll remember them for ever.

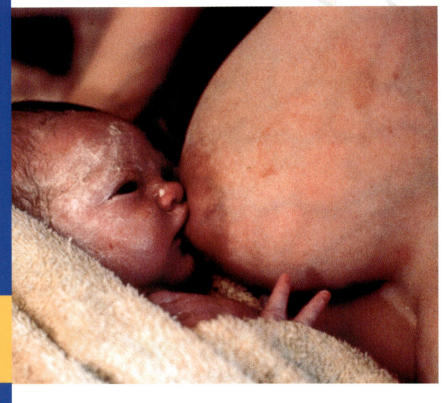

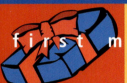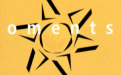

first moments

YOUR BABY'S FIRST BREASTFEED

You can offer the first breastfeed when your baby shows interest in feeding. Cuddle your baby in skin to skin contact (see page 83). When he begins to mouth and lick, it is a good time to offer the breast. Studies show that often newborn babies will 'crawl' to their mum's breast and position and attach themselves well at the breast if left in uninterrupted skin contact.

Caesarean birth

WHY IT'S DONE AND WHAT HAPPENS

A Caesarean birth means your baby is born by an operation. The surgeon makes an opening in your abdomen and then the uterus. In your notes, you may see it as LSCS, or LUSCS, which is the abbreviation for Lower Segment Caesarean Section, or Lower Uterine Segment Caesarean Section, or simply as CS (Caesarean Section).

You may know in advance that you will have a Caesarean section. You'll probably have it before you go into labour, so your appointment will be before your expected date of delivery. This advance planning is called an 'elective section'. Some women need a Caesarean section after going into labour and expecting to give birth

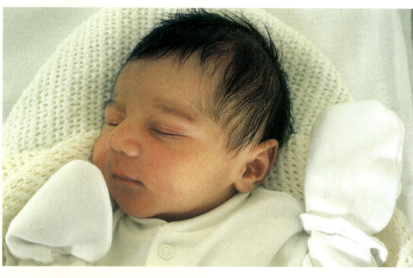

vaginally. This is called an emergency Caesarean section, although most cases are not as dramatic and last-minute as that sounds.

What happens to you

The operation is the same whatever type of anaesthetic you have. It's more common today to have an anaesthetic — a spinal or an epidural — which allows you to stay awake, though you should not feel any pain. Your partner or birth companion can usually be with you.

The surgeon first makes a cut at the base of your abdomen and then through the uterus, in a line just above your pubic hair.

You may feel some tugging when the baby is lifted out, sometimes by hand, sometimes with a pair of forceps. The baby's umbilical cord is cut and clamped, then he will be quickly checked over, and if all is well will be returned to you to hold. The placenta and membranes are delivered next, and then your uterus and abdomen are stitched. It only takes about 10 minutes to deliver the baby and about 30 minutes to stitch you afterwards.

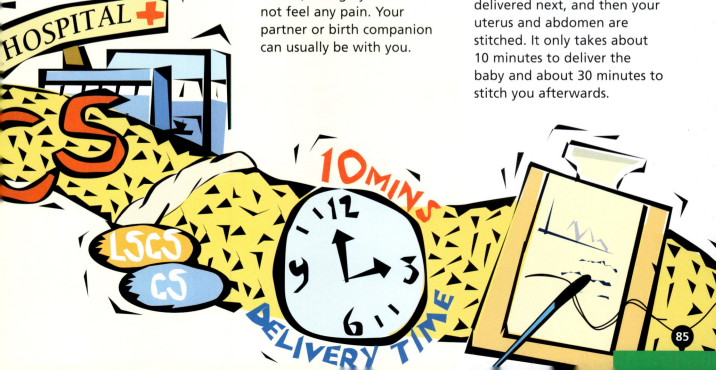

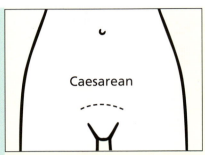

Usual place of cut

The reasons why you may decide on a Caesarean section include:

- you have a very low-lying placenta (called placenta praevia) which blocks your baby's way out

- multiple pregnancy — for some twins and almost always for triplets or more

- other complications, such as previous surgery on the vagina

- malpresentation — your baby is in a position which makes vaginal birth difficult or impossible.

Reasons for an emergency Caesarean section include:

- eclampsia or severe pre-eclampsia in the mother (see pages 55–56) means the pregnancy should end as soon as possible

- sudden onset of severe illness, such as kidney disease, or very high blood pressure

- the baby is in a poor or impossible position for birth ('malpresentation') or is too big to come out through the pelvis safely ('disproportion'). This may not have been apparent until labour had begun

- the baby is suffering from fetal distress (lack of oxygen) and labour hasn't progressed enough for a forceps or a ventouse delivery to be carried out safely

- your baby's head is too big for your pelvis, or your pelvis shape or size won't allow the baby to be born without major difficulty

- lack of progress in labour, when the contractions are weak and the cervix doesn't dilate.

Anaesthesia and Caesarean section

If you have a Caesarean section you will need total pain relief. Some women have a general anaesthetic, which means you are unconscious during the operation. Most women have an epidural or spinal anaesthetic. This completely numbs you from the site of the injection downwards, but allows you to remain fully awake and aware of everything but the pain.

You take time to recover from the effects of a general anaesthetic and there are more risks to the mother's health, and for this reason an epidural or spinal anaesthesia will usually be given. In some units, doctors administer a combined spinal and epidural which allows a top-up of anaesthetic when necessary.

AFTER YOUR SECTION

In the first days after your Caesarean section, you will feel very tired — probably more tired than after a vaginal birth — and you may have some pain, especially round your wound. You may suffer from intestinal wind, which is common after any abdominal operation. Laughing or coughing may hurt, too. The midwife will show you how to support your wound when you need to cough or laugh to avoid any pressure on your tummy. Wear large pants that come up to your waist, rather than briefs whose elastic may rub against your wound. You'll be offered pain-relief which is safe to take while breastfeeding.

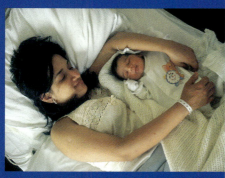

You may be fitted with a small drain which collects any blood that might otherwise pool under the wound. This is usually removed in a day or so. At first, an intravenous drip in your arm will replace lost fluids. You won't be able to get up to pass urine, and you will either have a catheter, or be helped to use a bedpan.

The stitches in your skin may simply dissolve or be removed later. Individual clips will also be removed.

Q. Will I need a Caesarean section if I have another baby?

A. Probably not, unless the reason for your Caesarean section occurs again, or if you produce a big baby and you have a small pelvis ('disproportion'). However, the diagnosis of disproportion is not always hard and fast, and you may want to ask for a second opinion.

If you go into labour, there is a slight risk that contractions may cause the scar on your uterus to start to tear. Although this is rare and can happen without warning, with proper care, this can be spotted before it becomes a problem.

Your feelings

Sometimes, women feel disappointed if they've had a Caesarean birth. To have the baby delivered 'for' you, can make you feel you have missed out on something essential. Then, if the baby is fine, you may feel guilty at being disappointed. Talk about these feelings with your partner, with your midwife, and with other mothers who have had Caesarean births. Understanding why you needed a Caesarean section can help you put the experience in perspective. Support organisations may help (see **Further help** at the back of this book).

Breastfeeding after a Caesarean section

If you have a Caesarean section, you can still cuddle your baby in close skin contact until she shows interest in feeding (see page 84).

You may need help in getting your baby comfortably positioned and attached in the first few days. Both you and your baby need to be comfortable, and you may find that raising your baby on a pillow across your lap avoids putting any pressure on your tummy. Or, you could try feeding while lying on your side. The 'football' hold is often found to be the most comfortable (the baby's legs between your arm and your body). Having a Caesarean section makes no difference to the way you produce milk.

The first days

CHANGES IN YOUR BABY

At first, your baby may look a little odd — even squashed and wrinkly, and possibly bluish on the hands and feet. Over the next few days, you'll notice the skin seems to smooth out a little, the head becomes rounder, and the whitish skin coating of vernix disappears.

Some babies sleep quite a lot in the first two or three days; others are quite alert and some want to be fed almost constantly. It is important to follow the baby's cues and feed on demand. Most babies do feed a lot at night, so sleep during the day if you can. Most units now recommend that babies stay with their mother 24 hours a day. This helps to establish feeding, and reduces the risk of infection. It is also important for security reasons.

CHECKS YOUR BABY MAY HAVE

In the first days after the birth, checks are offered to

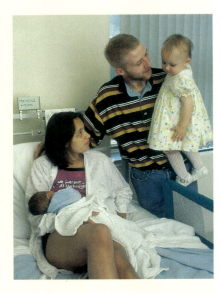

make sure your baby is healthy. The doctor or midwife will discuss them with you beforehand.

- **Heart.** If you are told your baby has an additional sound of the heart called a 'murmur', you may feel worried, but in fact the condition is very common. One estimate is that 50 per cent of babies have a heart murmur in the first week. Within a few weeks, most murmurs are not heard any more.

- **Congenital dislocation of the hip.** The doctor examines each hip joint to check that the head of the thigh bone (femur) moves as it should do within the socket for the femur at the hip, and that it doesn't slip out.

- **PKU — phenylketonuria.** A very rare (1 in 10,000) metabolic disorder. The blood spot test (formerly 'Guthrie' test) is carried out in the first week or so of life, usually after the fifth day, to check for this and some other conditions, such as congenital hypothyroidism (CPT). Your baby's heel is pricked, and several drops of blood are placed on a special card. This is then sent to the laboratory so the samples of blood can be tested. Ask the midwife what the tests will show.

- **Cystic fibrosis.** This is a condition which causes lung and digestive problems. The earlier treatment is started the better. From February 2003, all babies in Scotland will be screened for cystic fibrosis using the same sample of blood that is taken from the baby's heel for the blood spot test (see above).

- **Jaundice.** Checked usually just by observing the skin, which is yellowish if the baby has it. Many new babies have mild jaundice, caused by a substance called bilirubin still present in the blood.

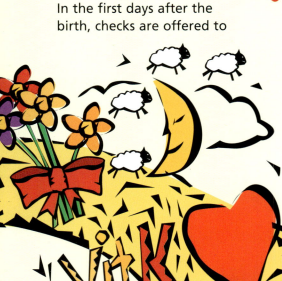

If the yellow colour of the skin doesn't go away, a blood check is done to see whether the jaundice is severe or not. Babies who remain jaundiced at 14 days should always be referred to a paediatrician for other investigations. There are other less common causes of jaundice which need to be ruled out. Most babies, however, are perfectly well.

- **Group B Streptococcus (Strep).** This is a germ carried by up to one-third of mothers, and it usually doesn't cause any harm. However, it can be passed to the baby during labour, and a few babies who catch it will become very sick if they are not treated. Babies who are infected will be given antibiotics to prevent them from becoming ill. In some areas, routine testing of mothers for Strep B is being considered. Ask your midwife about local policy and see **Further help** at the back of this book.

Reflexes checked for include:

- **the Moro or 'startle' reflex.** Your baby is supported on the tester's hand and forearm, and when the tester's hand is taken away from the head, the baby flings out her arms and legs, and then slowly settles back into position

- **the stepping response** comes if you hold your baby in a 'standing' position — both hands round the chest and facing away from you. Place one of the baby's feet on a hard surface (like a table). The leg of that foot extends, and the other leg moves forward, as if your baby was taking a step

- **the trunk incurvation reflex.** You will see this reflex if you stroke your baby's back firmly, following down the line of the spine. The baby's back will curve.

In most maternity units, Vitamin K for your baby is offered routinely in the labour ward, shortly after birth. This may prevent a rare condition called haemorrhagic disease of the newborn, when blood fails to clot. There are two ways of giving Vitamin K to your baby, orally (by mouth) or by injection.

Both ways offer protection to your baby. The difference is that if you choose 'by mouth' for your baby the dose will have to be repeated — twice for formula fed babies and at least three times for breastfed babies. This is because Vitamin K is already added to infant formula. You should be given as much information as you wish about this, and be asked for permission before Vitamin K is given.

FROM THE MOMENT OF BIRTH, YOUR BABY CAN:

- **see,** though focusing on objects more than about 25 cm (10 inches) away is difficult. The baby's eyes will follow your face, if you hold her up while you look at each other, and then turn your head

- **hear,** and be startled by loud noises. The baby seems to respond best to soft, light voices — the sort of tone most of us use instinctively when we are talking to a new baby

- **grasp,** seen if you touch the baby's palm. The toes will be flexed, too, if you stroke the soles of the baby's feet.

REGISTERING THE BIRTH

In Scotland, you must register your baby's birth within three weeks. The hospital or midwife notifies the local Child Health Unit within 36 hours, which in turn notifies the Registrar of births and your health visitor. You will receive a reminder if you don't register the birth within this time. If you are married to your baby's father, either of you can register your baby. If you are not married, and you want the baby's father to have his name on the certificate, then you need to go together to register the birth.

GOING HOME

Most first-time mothers stay in hospital for one or two nights. Your stay will be longer if you have a Caesarean section or if you or your baby need extra care. With second and subsequent babies you can often go home within a few hours or the next day if all is well. Try to organise as much help as possible at home.

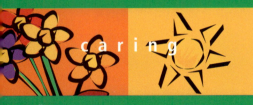

caring

Many women have mixed feelings about going home: relief and excitement mixed with nervousness. Before you leave hospital though, the midwives will have taught you the basics of baby care, feeding and safety. And the community midwife will continue to visit you at home to make sure that you and your baby are well, until your baby is at least 10 days old. After that, your health visitor will visit you both (see page 106).

If your baby was very small or premature, you will also probably stay in touch with the hospital paediatrician for a time, either directly or through a community neonatal nurse.

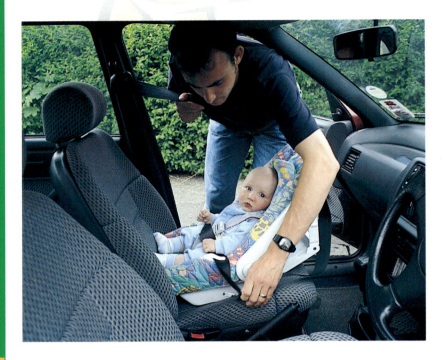

Remember car safety

You should use an appropriate child restraint on every journey including the one home from the hospital. It is dangerous to sit with your baby on your lap or in your arms.

A special baby seat can be used in either the front or back seat. It must be held in place by an adult seat belt. You can't use it with a seat belt that just goes over your lap.

If you have an airbag fitted on the passenger side your baby **must** travel in the back seat.

Learn how to fit and remove the seat before you use it with the baby. Some hospitals hire baby car seats. Some taxi services also supply a baby seat — ask for this special service if you ever use a taxi for you and your baby, and you don't have your own seat. (See also page 131.)

For safety, everyone in a vehicle must use a seat belt or child seat at all times when the vehicle is moving.

NEVER put your seat belt around yourself AND your baby

Feeding your baby

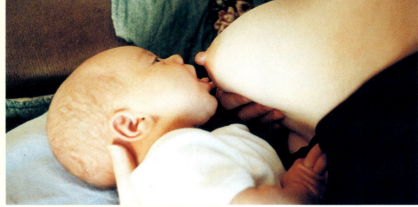

WHAT YOU NEED TO KNOW

Breastfeeding

Breast milk is the best food and drink for your baby. It is always high in quality, perfectly adapting itself to your baby's needs for the first four to six months of life. Breastfeeding is natural, but is something both mother and baby may have to learn to do. It helps if you feel confident, and those around you support you in your choice.

A good start

Immediately after the birth of your baby, the midwife will dry him well and then you can cuddle him next to you in close skin contact. The baby will enjoy hearing your heartbeat and getting to know your smell. Cuddling him next to you will stimulate your hormones and when he begins to mouth and lick you can encourage him to breastfeed. Some babies, if left in uninterrupted skin to skin contact with their mother after the birth, will crawl to the breast and position and attach themselves well at the breast.

When you and your baby are learning, these points may help.

Your baby's **position**:

- hold your baby close to you, turned towards you at the level of your breast
- his head, shoulders and body should be in a straight line so that he does not have to twist or turn his head
- his nostrils or top lip should be opposite your nipple.

Helping your baby **attach** well at the breast:

- position your baby as described with his nostrils or top lip opposite your nipple
- wait until his mouth is wide open (you can encourage him by brushing his bottom lip with your finger or your nipple)

- when his mouth is wide open bring the baby towards your breast. Aim your nipple towards his top lip or nostrils, so that his bottom lip is as far away from your nipple as possible when he attaches at the breast.

When you bring the baby towards your breast his head will be extended backwards slightly so that his chin comes into contact with your breast first. This is why it is so important not to hold the back of your baby's head as this will stop him from getting a large enough mouthful of the breast to attach correctly.

Signs that your baby is well positioned and attached:

- feeding is pain-free — after the first few seconds
- his sucking pattern changes — from vigorous sucking at the beginning to long deep sucks with pauses
- his chin will be touching the breast
- you may see the little muscle in front of his ear moving.

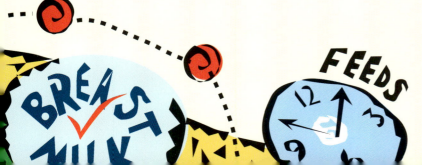

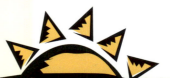

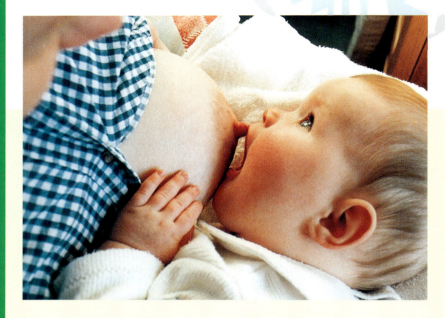

How it works

As the baby sucks and takes milk from the breasts, hormonal responses 'tell' your body to make more milk. The more you feed, the more milk you make — that's why mothers of twins make twice as much milk. Effective breastfeeding also stimulates the 'let-down' reflex which pushes milk stored deep inside the breast down into the ducts and out through the small outlets on the nipples.

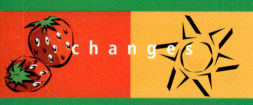

c h a n g e s

Later, you can encourage your baby into a routine, if you like. But in the early weeks, frequent, irregular feeds are normal for many babies. Long, frequent feeds without your baby ever seeming contented are a sign you and your baby need help. Sometimes small changes, perhaps to the way your baby is positioned and attached, make a real difference.

Changes in the early days

Your milk adapts to your baby's needs. The milk you produce in pregnancy and for the first few days after the birth is called colostrum. It is a highly-concentrated, straw-coloured fluid, rich in nutrients and antibodies which protect your baby. This is all your baby needs for now. Your milk 'comes in' between days two and five.

The first milk your baby gets at the start of the feed is called 'foremilk'. As the let-down reflex works, your breasts release fattier, calorie-rich 'hindmilk'. Your baby needs both foremilk and hindmilk to grow and to stay healthy. That's why it's best to leave it up to your baby to decide when she has had enough — don't take the baby off the breast after any particular time.

One 'side' or two?

Your baby may take one or both breasts at every feed. Let the baby stay on one breast as long as she likes, then offer the other. The baby may or may not take it. At the next feed, offer the second, or 'unused', breast first.

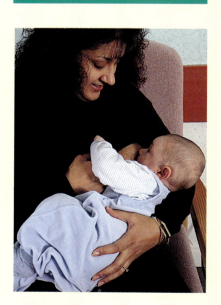

Q. **Do I need to drink or eat anything special when I am breastfeeding?**

A. No. Eat a balanced diet and drink according to thirst. You may be thirstier than usual, especially at first, but don't force yourself to drink more than you want to. Some women find they are a little hungrier, too. Don't avoid any foods unless you are certain they have caused a reaction in your baby. There's no evidence that any particular type of food will have more effect than any other. If you feel your baby reacts to something in your diet, speak to your midwife or health visitor or breastfeeding counsellor.

Some medication is best avoided by breastfeeding mothers. If your doctor or dentist prescribes something, say you are breastfeeding. Before taking any over-the-counter remedies, tell the pharmacist you are breastfeeding and check the packaging.

Alcohol in small amounts is not thought to be harmful but your baby's liver will take much longer than yours to break it down.

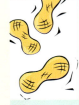

PEANUTS and foods containing peanut products should continue to be avoided if you or close relatives suffer from eczema, hayfever and asthma.

Breastfeeding protects your baby by building up immunity against a wide range of infections and conditions. Research has shown that breastfed babies have a reduced risk of:

- gastro-enteritis — vomiting and diarrhoea
- ear infections
- wheeze when breathing/asthma
- eczema, where this runs in the family
- developing diabetes in childhood
- urinary infections
- chest infections.

Breast milk has a special value for pre-term babies who are vulnerable to some potentially very dangerous conditions (such as neonatal necrotizing enterocolitis). Breast milk also ensures better brain development in pre-term babies.

Mothers who breastfeed have a reduced risk of:

- ovarian cancer
- pre-menopausal breast cancer.

When breastfeeding goes well, it's very enjoyable, and both mother and baby find it highly rewarding.

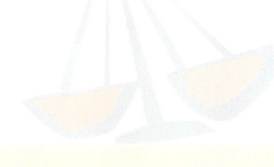

'I was never very keen on the idea of breastfeeding. I always knew I would find it awkward to feed in front of other people — I guessed I would feel embarrassed. I didn't have much confidence in my ability to produce enough milk, and at least with a bottle you can see how much milk the baby's getting. Then, I thought about the benefits, and promised myself I'd give it a fortnight.

'The first few days were difficult, and I shed a few tears. I was very sore, and my nipples cracked. But it got better, and I had a lot of support from the midwife who helped me to keep going and taught me how to get my baby latched on so my nipples healed. I practised feeding in ways that no one could actually see what I was doing — I wore T-shirts and tops that pulled up, and found the baby and my clothing hid my breast from view.

'Now he's four months, and I'm still doing it. It's easy now, and I keep thinking of all the work I've saved, not having to sterilise bottles and prepare feeds.'

Later breastfeeding

Mothers often say that breastfeeding gets easier after the first weeks. When it's going well you notice the convenience of it. If you have felt embarrassed at breastfeeding in front of others, that often disappears as your confidence grows. Your baby latches on quickly, feeds take less time, and your baby may feed less often. You can have time away from your baby when you need to, between feeds.

As time goes on, your milk is produced at the same time as your baby sucks, without a build-up of milk between feeds. If you notice your breasts feel softer and 'emptier' than before, it may mean that your supply is now responsive to the needs of your baby. You can carry on feeding as long as you want to. Once you have been breastfeeding for some months, your milk supply keeps going. One feed a day or less, which may be all a breastfeeding toddler takes, can be enough to maintain your supply.

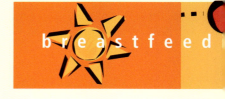

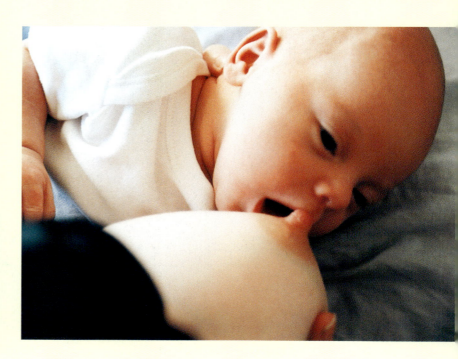

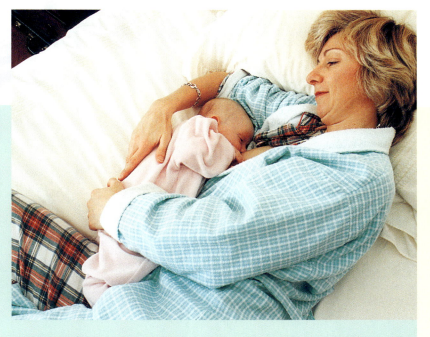

When breastfeeding isn't going well

Some women find breast-feeding difficult, particularly in the early days. But almost all difficulties can be solved. Many are avoidable in the first place, if the baby is attached and positioned at the breast correctly, and if allowed to feed when he wants.

Sore nipples: are almost always caused by poor positioning and attachment. Check, and if necessary, correct the way the baby takes the breast, and the baby's positioning and attachment. Sometimes, soreness is caused by thrush on the nipple. Both you and your baby need treatment from the doctor.

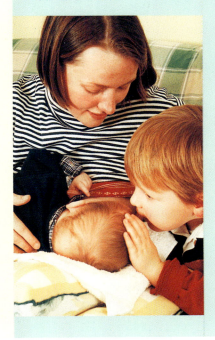

Blocked ducts and mastitis: this can happen when milk is not able to flow through one part of the breast. This means milk collects in the milk secretion and storage tissue (the alveoli). A blocked duct can be cleared by the baby feeding effectively. If the duct isn't cleared then mastitis can develop. Mastitis is an inflammation of the breast, with or without an infection. Symptoms are a lump, a red patch, pain on feeding and possibly flu-like feverishness in you. Continue feeding, but seek advice from a breastfeeding counsellor, health visitor or midwife. Very rarely your doctor may prescribe antibiotics, if there is an infection present.

Not enough milk: if you think you do not have enough milk, the first thing to do is check your baby's positioning and attachment (see page 91). If the baby is positioned and attached well, increasing the number of feeds will increase your supply. Let the baby feed for as long as he wants to.

Remember, almost every woman is able to make enough milk for her baby. Giving your baby bottles of water, formula or anything else may reduce your chances of successfully establishing breastfeeding. If bottle feeds fill your baby up, he will spend less time at the breast which can reduce the amount of milk you produce.

Read page 96 to reassure yourself that your baby is feeding well.

Breastfeeding help, friendship and support is on offer throughout Scotland in support groups. Or, contact one of the organisations that offer counselling to breastfeeding mothers. For information see page 151.

A word about weight gain

When you let your baby feed as often and as long as he wants, you can't see how much breast milk is being taken. The only 'proof' you have of growth is to look at weight gain on the growth chart. If it shows your baby is putting on less weight than expected, this can be worrying for you. But remember, weight charts can be misleading, as they were developed from studying the growth of bottle-fed babies, and also may not apply to all cultures.

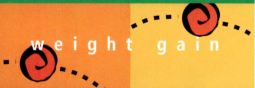

Weight is only one indicator of a baby's progress. There are others. For example, an alert, healthy baby, who appears content and satisfied after most feeds, and who usually manages to get attached to the breast without a fuss, is giving you signs that breastfeeding is working well.

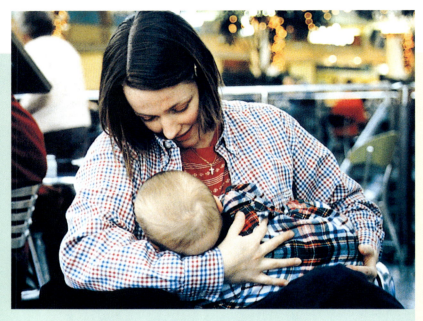

How do you know your baby is feeding well?

Healthy, well-nourished, breastfed babies:

- manage to get attached to the breast without any fuss at most feeds

- have 5–6 wet nappies every day

- pass soft, yellow stools after the first few days. The occasional green stool is not usually significant. Most breastfed babies pass several stools a day at first, then after a few weeks they may go several days between bowel movements, though frequent motions are also normal. (You can get more information about the way your baby's stools change in the first days on page 112.)

- develop as expected (for instance, smiling by about six weeks).

Note: your baby should be weighed without clothing or a nappy every time.

Watch for your baby sucking and swallowing while on your breast. At the start of the feed he may suck quickly, then he may continue more rhythmically and deeply. He may pause occasionally, and then continue. After a time, he may come off the breast, full and looking 'zonked'!

Q. Is it possible to mix breastfeeding with bottle feeding?

A. It's true that some mothers do — but giving bottles early interferes with the establishment of successful breastfeeding, and the experience of many breastfeeding specialists suggests that the later you leave mixing breast and bottle, the better.

However, once breastfeeding is well established — say, after six or seven weeks — some mothers find the occasional bottle makes no long-term difference to their supply. Working mothers find they can breastfeed twice a day in the week, and fully at weekends, and their body adjusts to these different demands. Some babies are reluctant to take a bottle from their mothers, but tolerate it if it's given by someone else.

Q. Can I start to breastfeed after a period of bottle feeding?

A. Yes, but the sooner you switch, the better. In the first days, you produce milk whether or not your baby has come to the breast at all. The milk goes away if the supply isn't stimulated by the baby's sucking, but it can come back if it is stimulated again. This is known as 'relactation'. It is physically possible to relactate, but you need a cooperative baby who is willing to suck, even when there is very little milk.

There are special breastfeeding aids to help you in this situation which supply formula milk down a tube attached to your nipple, so the baby gets rewarded for sucking. Breastfeeding counsellors, midwives and health visitors can give you more information.

Working and breastfeeding

Many mothers enjoy keeping up the closeness of breastfeeding after their return to work, and the health benefits of breast-feeding are worth the extra organisation you need to ensure it's possible (see page 93). Your employer may have a duty to help you continue, by providing facilities to express and store your milk and avoiding extending your hours or travelling time in ways that might prevent you breastfeeding. The Maternity Alliance has information for you and your employer on this issue (see page 155). Here are your main options.

- Leave expressed breast milk (EBM — see over the page) for your baby. As a rough guide, a baby under three months will take 100–120 ml of expressed breast milk per feed, and a baby over three months will take 150–200 ml (5–7 fluid ounces) per feed. But this is very general — after you have done it a few times, you'll soon become good at knowing what your baby is likely to need.

- Breastfeed your baby when you're together, and leave formula when you're apart. You will probably need to express at work at first, to keep yourself comfortable, but your body soon adapts. You can even fully breastfeed at weekends.

- Babies from five or six months on can have EBM or formula in a cup when you're not there (that way, there's no need to get them used to a bottle).

A separate booklet *Breastfeeding and Returning to Work* is available from your midwife or health visitor.

Expressing your milk

This means removing the milk from your breasts by hand or with a special hand pump (available from chemists or baby stores) — your midwife, health visitor or a breastfeeding counsellor can explain what to do. Electric breast pumps can be hired from breastfeeding support organisations.

By hand

- Firstly, you need to find where your milk-collecting ducts are on your breasts. Feel down your breast until you feel the texture changing. The ducts are often found at the edge of the areola or about three-quarters of an inch from the nipple but their position varies from woman to woman, therefore you need to feel your breast to find where your own are situated. Some women say that the milk-collecting ducts feel like small elongated peas.
- Place the flat of your thumb and finger over the milk-collecting ducts above and below your nipple as shown in the picture.
- Gently push your breast back towards the chest wall.
- Gently squeeze your

thumb and finger together without sliding them over your skin.
- Release the pressure and repeat the process building up into a rhythm (your finger and thumb should remain in the same position).

At first you will produce drips of milk and then jets of milk. When the jets return to drips it is important that you repeat the process with your fingers over a different set of milk-collecting ducts so that you express milk from other lobes of the breast. You can do this by rotating your fingers around your breast.

Sometimes it helps if you stroke your breast gently or massage it to stimulate the hormones before you start expressing. Many women find that with practice they can express from both breasts at the same time.

Breast milk should always be expressed into a sterilised container.

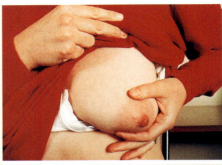

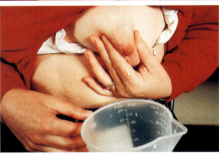

Storing your milk

The most up-to-date advice is that milk can be kept in the fridge for up to five days. EBM can also be frozen for up to six months. Your fridge and freezer need to be clean and the temperature reliable. You can also store and transport EBM in a cool-bag until you get home — that's useful if you are expressing at work and don't have a fridge you can use there.

The book, *Off to a Good Start: All you need to know about breastfeeding your baby,* is available from your midwife or health visitor.

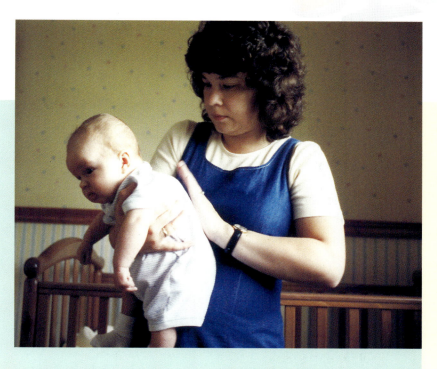

Bottle feeding

Baby formula milk is used instead of breast milk, if a mother doesn't breastfeed. Babies should have only baby formula milk, not ordinary pasteurised cow's milk, until the age of one year (though pasteurised whole cow's milk can be used in cooking from six months).

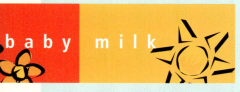

Cow's milk products (eg yoghurts, fromage frais and custards) can be used in weaning after six months.

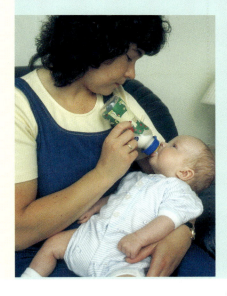

Formula milk is usually based on cow's milk which has been modified to meet babies' specific nutritional needs. For babies who cannot tolerate cow's milk (eg in cases of lactose intolerance, cow's milk sensitivity and galactosaemia), hydrolysed protein formulas are available and can be prescribed. These are preferable to soya-based formulas which may pose a long-term risk to infants because of their high phytoestrogen content.

Formula milk is sold in cans or packets, in powdered or granule form, to be mixed with water. Ready-to-feed formula is also sold in cartons. It's more expensive than dried formula.

Follow-on milks are infant formulas suitable for older babies (the recommended minimum age in the UK is six months). They have no advantage over breast milk or ordinary infant formula.

Q. Why is it so important to sterilise?

A. Warm milk is a breeding ground for harmful germs. A fully bottle-fed baby doesn't get the natural protection against infection in breast milk, so it's essential you sterilise equipment to minimise the risk. Ask your health visitor for advice about how long to do it for, but the usual advice is to sterilise all your baby's feeding equipment until he is six months, and then to carry on doing so with his milk feeding equipment for a year.

Q. Breastfeeding was such a struggle, and I changed to formula. But I feel guilty now.

A. Mothers can feel very sad and disappointed if breastfeeding doesn't work out. It can help to work out what went wrong. Perhaps you weren't able to get him on the breast in a way that got your milk supply off to a good start. Maybe you got poor information and support. Talking things over with a breastfeeding counsellor can help to reassure you that it wasn't your fault, and give you confidence if you have another baby.

What you need to bottle feed

- At least six 200 ml bottles, teats and bottle covers.
- Formula milk.
- Bottle brush, teat brush.
- Sterilising equipment.

All feeding equipment must be kept clean, to protect your baby against infection. Wash everything after use in hot soapy water, and use the brushes to make sure all deposits are removed. If you don't use a teat brush, turn teats inside out to clean them. Rinse everything in clear water and then sterilise.

Sterilise:

- by boiling the equipment in a covered pan for at least 10 minutes, making sure there is no air trapped in the bottles or teats
- by using a chemical sterilising solution (follow the manufacturer's instructions). Leave in the solution for at least 30 minutes. Make up a fresh solution every 24 hours
- by steaming, in a special steam steriliser
- by using a sterilising unit made for the microwave oven.

Always wash your hands before removing the equipment. If you wish to rinse the equipment before using, use boiled cooled water.

Making up a feed

If you have lead plumbing in your house, or leading to your house, see the important note on page 128.

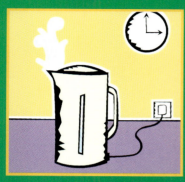

1. Boil a kettle with fresh tap water. Allow it to cool.

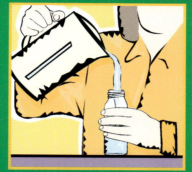

2. Wash your hands thoroughly. Stand the bottle on a clean surface. Pour in the correct amount of water.

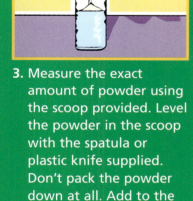

3. Measure the exact amount of powder using the scoop provided. Level the powder in the scoop with the spatula or plastic knife supplied. Don't pack the powder down at all. Add to the water. Replace disc, teat and cover.

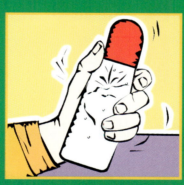

4. Shake well until all the powder has dissolved.

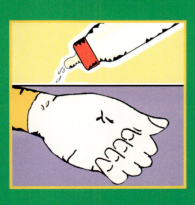

5. The feed should be warm when you give it to your baby. Check the temperature by dripping a little on to the inside of your wrist — it should feel neither warm nor cold. You can cool it by running the bottle under the cold tap.

Note: always get rid of unused milk at the end of every feed. If you have made up several bottles at a time, get rid of any that are unused after 24 hours.

Making up feeds in advance

You can keep bottles in the fridge for 24 hours. Cover the teats with bottle covers, or leave the teats off and cover the bottle with the disc. Warm the milk by standing the bottle in a jug of hot water or in a special bottle warmer. Never use the microwave oven — it creates random hot spots which could scald your baby's mouth.

Always use the correct proportions of water to powder. The amount of made-up milk suggested on the pack is only a guide. Follow your baby's appetite.

Don't use soya formula without medical advice.

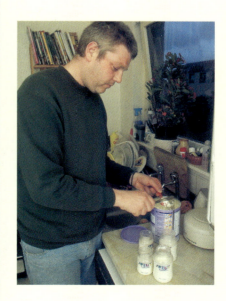

Your life after the birth

CHANGES YOU CAN EXPECT

Immediately after the birth, your tummy will look saggy and soft. Most women regain their pre-pregnancy weight and shape simply by eating normally — though you may never look **exactly** the same. Exercise may speed things up, and it's important to do the pelvic floor exercises to restore tone to this area (see page 103). If you have had a Caesarean section or split abdominal muscle some exercises may not be suitable for you — ask your midwife or an obstetric physiotherapist.

The uterus still contracts in the days after birth, as it goes back to its pre-pregnancy size. You may sometimes feel these contractions (known as 'afterpains'). If you find them too painful (not everyone does) ask the midwife or GP which painkillers are safe to take.

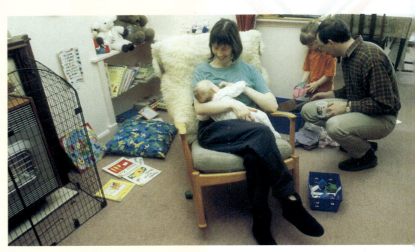

Your breasts may increase in size and feel more tender when your milk comes in (see page 92). This is a result of the increase in milk, blood and lymph in the breast tissue.

Vaginal discharge (lochia) after childbirth is a mix of blood and other material squeezed out of the uterus. At first it's bright red, then pinkish brown, through to cream. It's quite heavy at first and you will need several changes of sanitary pads a day (tampons are not recommended, because of the risk of infection). During the first 24 hours some women find disposable nappies more effective than sanitary pads.

After the first week it slows down a lot, but you may find it lasts three or four weeks before finally disappearing. Get medical advice if you start to lose fresh red blood when your bleeding has previously been brown, or if the discharge is smelly, or if you have abdominal pain, or a temperature. However, some fresh red blood loss is normal after a breastfeed.

Constipation for a couple of days is very common after childbirth. Help yourself by drinking plenty of fluids and eating high-fibre foods, including fresh fruit and vegetables.

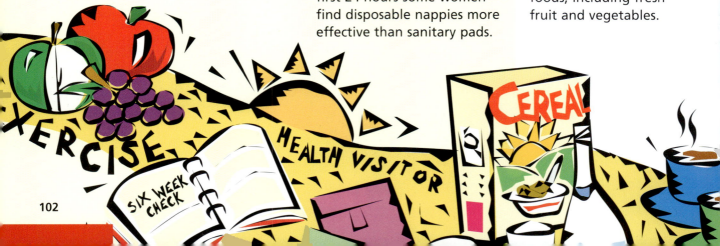

The six-week postnatal check

Around six weeks after the birth, you'll be invited to see either your GP, the community midwife, or a doctor at the unit where your baby was born.

This is a routine assessment, done to make sure you are returning to normal physically, and that if you're not, any problems can be dealt with. It's also an opportunity to ask you how you feel, and to answer any questions you may have. You can also talk about contraception at this check-up if you want.

The doctor may suggest doing an internal examination, and palpate your abdomen, to make sure the uterus has returned to its pre-pregnancy size. If you don't feel ready for this, say so.

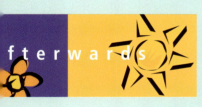

I felt this pressure to get back to normal — and I wanted some time and space to myself. I found the baby just totally overwhelming — I couldn't stop being worried about her, and scared I was doing everything wrong.'

'Baby blues'

'Postnatal blues' or 'baby blues' is a very common feeling of tearfulness, around two or three days after the birth. It's rather like coming down to earth after the 'high' of giving birth. It could also be hormonal, as this is about the time the mature milk 'comes in'. You may find yourself weeping, and feeling 'at sea' among your new emotions. It usually passes after a day or so, but you will need extra support while it lasts (see also pages 107–109 on postnatal depression).

Pelvic floor exercises

Pelvic floor exercises can help you regain the tone in these important muscles. They help prevent the stress incontinence (see page 52) that can occur after childbirth (causing you to leak a few drops of urine when you cough, laugh or run). You may not feel you have any control over your pelvic floor muscles immediately after birth and for the next couple of days.

Remember, the more often you do them, the better! You'll be taught how to do them in pregnancy or after birth by a midwife or a physiotherapist. Start in the first days after the birth, and aim for four or five sets of 10 or 12 exercises each day. You can do them at any time — in fact it's a good idea to get into the habit of doing them every day of your life, and to make them a part

of your routine. It may be helpful to form the habit by remembering to do them **after** you pass urine each time.

Do them gently at first.

1. **Imagine you are trying to stop yourself passing urine. Tighten your front passage to prevent leaking.**

2. **Relax slowly, as you breathe out.**

3. **Repeat.**

If your pelvic floor muscles are weak you may find this quite difficult at first. With frequent practice, though, you will soon improve. If you don't, see your GP. To check if your muscles are effective, try stopping the passage of urine in mid-stream. Do not do this too often, just once every few weeks will be enough.

YOUR RELATIONSHIPS, YOUR LIFE

Many things change after the birth. You may feel you have begun a whole new phase in your life, yet all the world's attention seems to be on your baby's needs, and not your own. Your greatest needs will include time, and adult support and conversation. You may feel your life has been taken over by the baby. If anyone offers to help, think of something they can do — or they may never ask again! Most people are delighted to think they can do you a small favour, and enjoy sharing in the upheaval a new baby brings.

Your partner

Trust your partner to care for the baby, and share your pleasures and anxieties. Spend time alone, if you can, as a couple — though this may not be easy to achieve for a while!

Your family and friends

Offers of help and support may be welcome, but don't feel you have to entertain them when they visit. If you find it tiring to see people, don't be afraid to ask visitors to come another time, or else arrange to visit them.

'People relate to you differently when you've had a baby. I feel my friends are more interested in the baby than me! I suppose they could be thinking "Maybe I'll be next".'

'My main memory of those first few weeks was being tired — every night was broken, usually more than once. Sometimes, the crying went on for hours. That wears you down. It was great when we could see he was growing out of it. You feel you must be doing something wrong, even when people tell you you're not.'

(Partner)

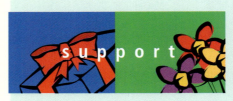

'It took a while to get close to the baby. It was great after she was born, and I know I loved her, but I don't think I had what you might call a "relationship" with her for ages. I only really started to enjoy her when she was a few months old, and showed me that she enjoyed being with me ... she gets excited when she hears me come in, and holds her arms out to me to be picked up. I love that!'

(Partner)

Making new friends

In most areas there are groups of other parents whose support and friendship can be a great help. If you're shy, it can be hard to break into these networks, so you may need to be quite brave and patient. Some organisations have coffee groups, or drop-in centres, or toddler clubs. Ring up to check on time and place of a meeting. Say who you are, ask who they are, and then ask for them by name when you get there. At least that way, you'll feel you know (or sort of know) someone. Don't be put off if you've picked a group that seems like a clique. That does happen, unfortunately. Either try again, or try another group.

Your health visitor will know of other people you can meet, and put you in touch, and will be a good source of information about different clubs. A health visitor can help you start your own group, if there's nothing to suit you.

Q. Does breastfeeding act as a contraceptive?

A. Breastfeeding may affect ovulation, which means you are less likely to produce an egg. You are less likely to conceive, and your periods are suppressed.

One method of contraception uses the fact that breastfeeding (lactation) means you may not menstruate ('amenorrhoea' means no menstruation). It is called the 'lactational amenorrhoea' method of family planning.

If you want to use this method as a contraceptive, speak to a counsellor or a doctor. For this to work you need to breastfeed exclusively and often, without giving any bottles, including through the night. **Even so, there is no guarantee you won't conceive using this method. If you want to be sure of avoiding a pregnancy, you need to use another form of contraception.** Ovulation happens before menstruation, so your fertility can return without you realising.

Some women don't menstruate when they are breastfeeding — even when the baby is older, and well-established on solid food, perhaps feeding only once or twice a day. Other women find their periods return when their baby starts to space feeds, or begins taking anything other than breast milk. Some start as early as a few weeks after the birth.

Sex after childbirth

You may be asked about contraception choices very soon after the birth — maybe when sex is absolutely the very last thing on your mind! Health professionals raise the topic so that you have time to think about this before the decision becomes more pressing. You can get advice at any time, though, from your doctor, health visitor or family planning clinic.

If you are breastfeeding, you'll be advised to avoid the combined pill — the sort that contains oestrogen and progesterone. This is because oestrogen may reduce the amount of milk you produce. The progesterone-only pill (sometimes known as the mini-pill) is more suitable (see also 'Family Planning' in the **Further help** section).

If you resume intercourse, you should start using your chosen method of contraception within four weeks of the birth to ensure protection. If you use a diaphragm or a cap, you should get it checked, to make sure it still fits (the cervix can change size and shape slightly after birth).

For many women a condom may be the simplest choice for the early weeks after childbirth.

If sex hurts, see your doctor about this. If you feel too 'dry' for sex, use a lubricant like KY Jelly. This is safe to use with a condom or diaphragm, as oil-based lubricants can damage them.

How soon should you, or can you, start making love after the birth — and what if you don't want to?

Physically, there's no reason why you shouldn't make love as soon as the lochia (discharge) has ceased and any cut or tear in the perineum has healed (before then, there may be a risk of infection). In practice, you may want to wait longer — both men and women vary a lot in how soon they want to resume their sex life. Remember, either or both of you may just feel too tired for sex — this is quite normal.

Be patient with yourselves. If you are breastfeeding, your breasts and nipples may be tender at first. If you've been stitched, you may feel bruised and battered for a while. Emotionally, a long, tiring or difficult labour can make you feel less ready to share your body.

Keep in physical and emotional touch with each other. Arrange special times for love-making — you can't be as spontaneous as you were, when you have a baby who may need your attention at any time.

Even if you can't, or don't want to, make love properly or fully, you can show your love for each other in many different, sensual ways — share a special dinner (or take-away) and leave the washing-up until the next day; give each other a sensuous massage.

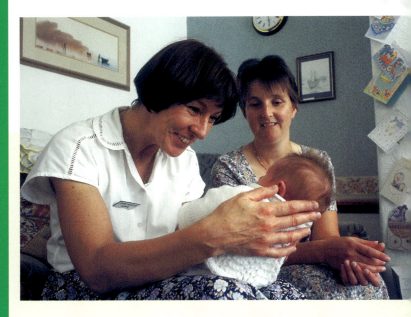

SUPPORT FOR YOU AND YOUR BABY

The midwife is responsible for your care for the first 10 days after the birth, and can extend this for longer, if needed. In practice, hospital midwives transfer your care to the community, and one or more community midwives will visit you at home after you have left hospital. The schedule of visits can be discussed between you and the midwife.

Very often the midwife transfers your care to the health visitor after the tenth day. Your health visitor will visit you and your baby soon after. One of the health visitor's responsibilities is to care for families with children under five (see also pages 37 and 122).

You should have a phone number to call a midwife and a health visitor if you need help outside normal working hours. Your health visitor will give you a number to call. She will also tell you about the baby clinic, and when you can bring your baby for immunisations. She may give you a child health record, a booklet for keeping information about your baby's growth, health, immunisations, and so on.

If you had a difficult birth, you may find yourself thinking about it a lot, perhaps wondering why it happened. It can help to talk about it with someone who understands pregnancy and childbirth, and who can explain some of the technical side to you. You, your GP or your midwife or health visitor can get hold of your notes if you don't have them, and you can go through the written account together.

Postnatal depression

WHY ARE SOME WOMEN DEPRESSED AFTER CHILDBIRTH?

Postnatal depression (PND) is quite common in the weeks and months after childbirth, and the causes of it are not yet fully understood. There may be several different reasons why it happens, and it may take different forms. For example, one of the reasons may be the pressures on new mothers to be 'back to normal' soon after the birth, and to feel capable and confident. When a mother doesn't feel that way, she often feels guilty and inadequate. Some mothers feel isolated with a new baby. They may find it hard to make new friends and contacts, and loneliness can be a major problem.

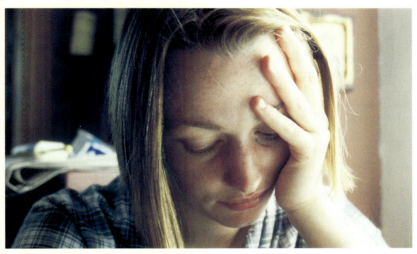

The mothers they do see may seem to be 'coping' better — and that can make them feel worse.

Mothers are expected to love their babies straight away, and although most mothers find these feelings grow and become more intense, they may not be there at the start of motherhood. Instead, there's a feeling of indifference, and guilt and sadness at feeling that way.

Some experts believe there may be a hormonal cause to PND, and that women who suffer from it can be helped with hormone treatment.

Mothers sometimes try to hide how they feel. They have high expectations of themselves and blame themselves for not matching up to them. It's as if the mother with PND feels that everyone else seems to be doing okay, and if she isn't, then it has to be her fault.

PND is different from the so-called 'baby blues' detailed on page 103. If you continue to feel low 10 days or more after the birth, then speak to a health professional.

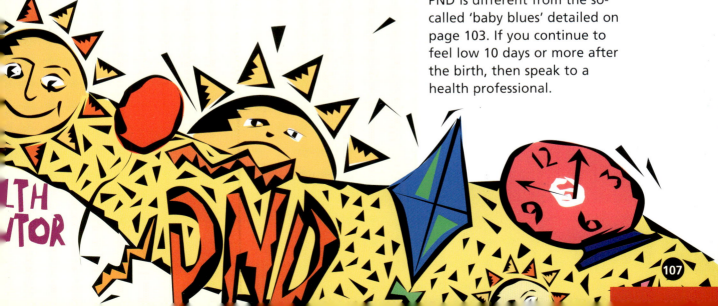

You may have PND if you have some of the following symptoms:

- time passes you by sometimes — you can look at the clock and wonder where the last two hours went

- you wake up each morning feeling exhausted, as if you haven't had any sleep

- you find you laugh and smile less than you used to

- you find it hard to concentrate, or organise simple tasks

- you feel a failure

- it's hard for you to see 'the funny side' of things

- you sometimes feel numb, as if feelings and experiences don't reach you

- simple tasks may require enormous effort

- you find yourself crying, or feeling tearful, for small things, or for no reason at all

- you feel you can only be yourself with your partner, and sometimes not even then.

Help is available. It may be that the most important part of treatment for PND involves friendship and social support. Health visitors in particular have been active in offering one-to-one support for depressed mothers, and by setting up groups where new mothers with PND (as well as those who are lonely, or bored, or isolated) can find help from getting to know each other, and talking in an understanding environment about their situation.

Your doctor may prescribe anti-depressants. Some anti-depressants are considered to be best avoided when breastfeeding. However, not all experts agree about the implications of this.

The medication may reach the milk, but switching to formula may have a greater effect on the baby's long-term health. There are no clear-cut answers to this question, so you should discuss your options with your doctor.

Psychotherapy has also been shown to help. This involves talking to a therapist about the experience of being a mother and what went on in your own childhood and afterwards, too. Sometimes, motherhood touches parts of us that we had forgotten about, or hidden away. It's thought that dealing with these unresolved emotions can help with PND.

The important point to remember is that PND is curable. It is just not worth suffering in silence. If you think you may need help, speak to your health visitor, midwife or doctor.

'I didn't even know I had postnatal depression ... hard to believe now. I had heard of PND, of course, and my cousin had suffered from it, too. But when it came to my own feelings, I knew I just didn't feel right, without really putting a label on myself. I just felt I wasn't a very good mother, that Joseph was a difficult, wakeful baby, and too much for me to cope with. I know I had to drag myself through the day, and that a lot of energy went on trying to act "normal". In the end, it was my health visitor who encouraged me to go for help. She recognised that things weren't as they should be, and we talked about what I felt and so on. My doctor helped me, though it took a few months before I felt I was better.'

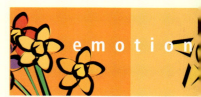

emotion

PUERPERAL PSYCHOSIS

Very occasionally, a mother can suffer a severe form of mental illness called puerperal psychosis. It happens to between 1 and 2 in every 1000 new mothers. It's different from PND, and needs different treatment.

Mothers with this illness can lose touch with reality at times. Typically, they have strange ideas, and/or hallucinations. They may be very energetic or else extremely down. It's soon obvious to anyone close to them that they are ill. (This is different from postnatal depression, where it's possible to hide the symptoms for a long time.)

Psychiatric treatment is needed, and the mother may be admitted into hospital, perhaps with her baby if there are the facilities for the baby to be cared for as well.

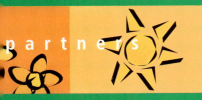

partners

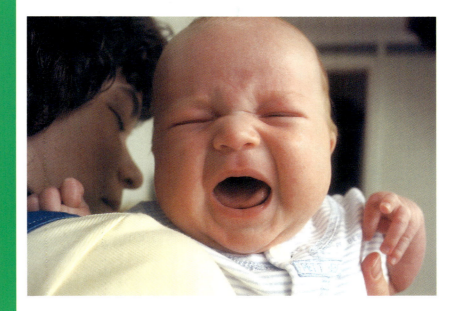

PARTNERS AND POSTNATAL DEPRESSION

Partners are especially important for women going through postnatal depression. The partner may be the only person a depressed woman can be herself with — and so gets the full impact of her distress. Partners may be angry and need help themselves. Their love and encouragement are essential for recovery, and their insistence on getting help may be the first step on that path. It may help a woman if she has her partner with her when she goes to seek treatment. A partner may be better at remembering what was said during the consultation, to remind her later.

Recent research has suggested that men, too, can suffer depression after they become fathers. It's not yet fully understood, but men may benefit from counselling and other forms of therapy, too. Speak to your doctor.

Routine care

BATHING, NAPPY CHANGING, CLOTHING

Bathing your baby the first few times can be quite daunting — your baby is so small and wriggly, and it's natural to feel scared you'll do something wrong. You'll become more confident as the weeks go by.

'Top and tail' your baby

A daily or twice-daily 'top and tail' is a quick alternative to a bath for a young baby. You need:

- cotton wool or two soft, clean cloths

- bowl of warm water

- a fresh nappy and clean clothes if necessary

- a bin or bucket for waste.

Wash your hands. Undress your baby on her back and leave the nappy on.

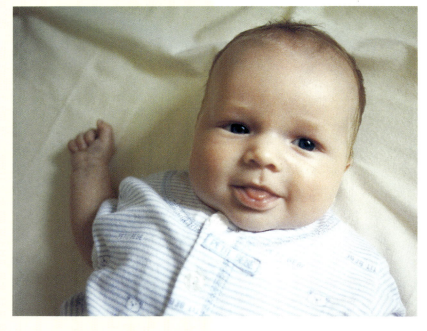

A very new baby may be more comfortable if wrapped in a towel to stay warm.

Wipe your baby's face, neck and ears. Dry with cotton wool or the other cloth, or a towel.

Now wipe the underarms and the hands. Dry.

Take off the nappy. For a new baby, wash any dried discharge that may have come from the cord stump. Wash the bottom and the genitals well. Wipe girls with a clean wet cloth from front to back. Pat dry. Use a protective cream to prevent nappy rash if you wish.

Replace the nappy and dress your baby.

> Use plain water, or unscented toiletries made for babies, to keep your baby clean. In the first weeks, most babies don't need anything on their skin. The skin produces its own protection, which can be affected by the use of scented or harsh toiletries.

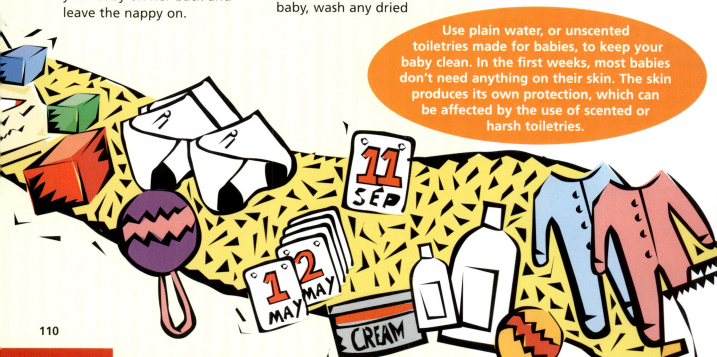

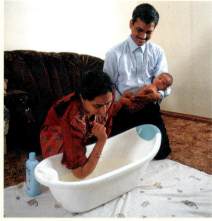
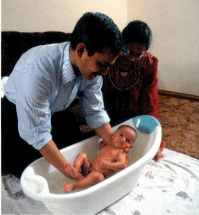
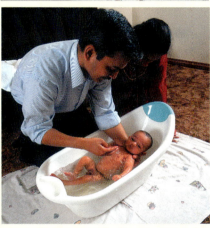
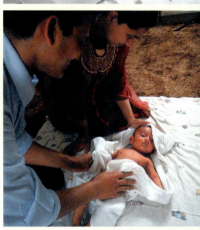

questions & answered

Q. How do I wash my baby's hair?

A. If your baby doesn't have much hair, you need only rinse the scalp during the bath, pouring some water over it with your hand or a jug. Longer-haired babies may need a tiny drop of mild shampoo on wet hair, lathered and rinsed off. To wash your baby's hair you can support the head and shoulders as she lies in the bath, and pour the water over with your other hand. Alternatively, you can wrap your baby in a towel and hold her over the bath with one hand, using your other hand to wash.

If your baby has cradle cap — greasy, crusty deposits on the scalp — you can rub in baby or vegetable oil to loosen this, and rinse off.

Bathing

Here's what to do — and all you'll need to know!

- Choose a warm, draught-free room.

- Make sure you have everything you need within reach. **Never leave a baby or a toddler alone in the bath, even for a few seconds, as there is a risk of drowning.** If you need to get something, or answer the phone, take your baby with you, wrapped in a towel.

- Whether you're using a baby bath, or the big bath, put cold water in first and then hot. Test the temperature with your elbow. It should feel comfortably warm.

- Lower your baby into the water, on her back, supporting the head and shoulders on your hand and forearm.

- Use your free hand to wet your baby's body and rub over the skin gently with a clean cloth.

- You can use a mild soap or baby bath liquid if you like, but it's not really necessary in the first few weeks.

- Dry your baby in a large absorbent towel and then dress.

Note: you can take your baby into the bath with you, as long as the water isn't too hot. You will need someone to hand you the baby after you get in, and to take the baby from you while you get out.

Nappies

Throw-away nappies are convenient, but expensive compared to washable nappies (even with the cost of washing). They are also hard to get rid of. Green campaigners say they take up space in landfill rubbish sites, take many years to rot down, and are a health hazard if dumped. If you want to use cotton, washable nappies, you can either wash and dry them at home yourself, or use a nappy laundry service, where there is one. The service takes away your dirty nappies and swaps them for clean ones.

Your baby's stools

At first your baby's stools are dark green or blackish, and sticky. This is known as meconium. They change over the first few days to a soft-textured yellow. Bottle-fed babies' stools may be more formed, and a pale brown colour. Some formula milks make the stools greenish. The occasional green stool in a breastfed baby does not matter.

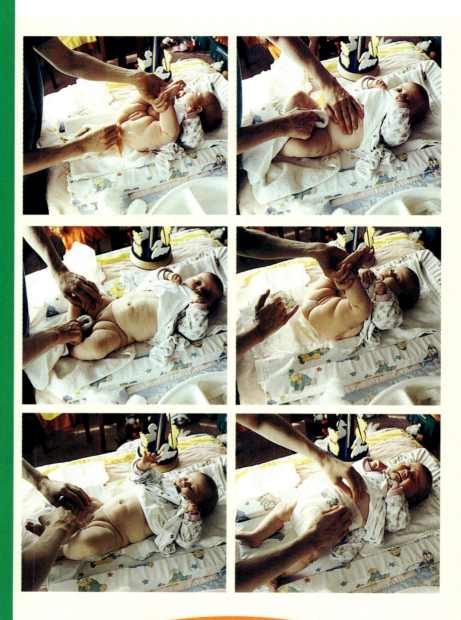

Nappy rash affects many babies. The symptoms are redness or soreness in the nappy area. Dirty nappies should be changed as soon as possible. Clean and dry your baby's bottom carefully to help prevent nappy rash. You can also try leaving your baby to kick without a nappy for a short period. Sometimes a rash can get infected, perhaps with thrush. See your health visitor or your doctor.

Clothing — some of the things your child will need

When your baby is young, keep clothing simple with designs that make for easy nappy changing (for example, front-fastening, and poppers up the inside of the legs).

Here's a suggested minimum that will see your baby through the first three months:

- five all-in-one stretchsuits
- five vests
- three cardigans or matinee jackets
- shawl
- bedding for pram — four sheets, two blankets
- bedding for crib/cot — four sheets, two blankets
- hat — warm for winter baby, sunhat for a summer baby
- nappies
- two towels, two washcloths, six cloths (in muslin or soft cotton) for wiping after and between feeds.

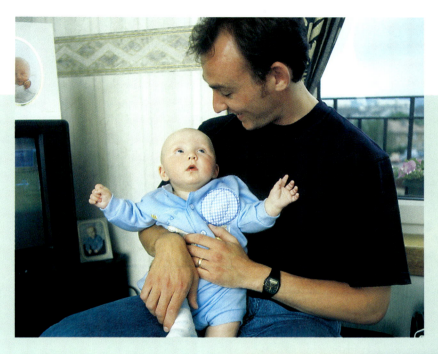

After three months, your baby will probably have grown out of some clothes. As he moves around more, you will need socks, and an outer garment, since less time will be spent in the cot or pram. The baby will need nightclothes, too, as you will probably develop an evening routine of a bath followed by bed. Bibs are essential when your baby starts solid food — you may need about a dozen.

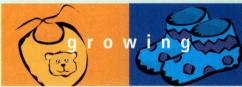

growing

Toddlers need several sets of clothes, as they dirty their clothes very quickly. Once your child is walking outside, he needs shoes. Feet should be measured for length and width, and checked for fitting every three to four months. Good shoe shops won't mind you checking on this, without buying new shoes. Make sure socks fit properly, too.

BABY EQUIPMENT

Later equipment

Most babies grow out of their baby cribs by about three months, so you will need a full-size cot from then on. From about six months, you may need a high chair.

Your child will probably move from a cot to a bed at between two and three years old (see page 117).

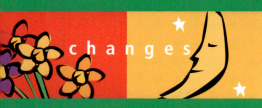

c h a n g e s

Baby slings

These can generally be used from birth (front slings). They allow you to carry your baby close to you, while leaving your hands and arms free. Back packs are designed for older babies who can support their head and neck. You and your partner should try on a few different models before you decide what to buy.

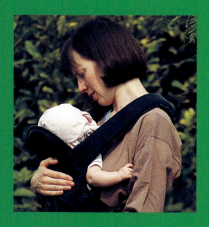

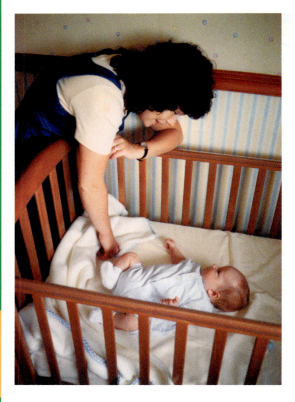

Items for the pram and/or lie-back pushchair

- In a pram, your baby needs one or two layers of lightweight blanket on top in cold weather, waterproof protection from the rain, and a sheet underneath. More layers are needed in a lightweight pushchair, and more if the weather is exceptionally cold. A fabric pushchair, or one which is low to the ground, will be cosier with a blanket underneath your baby as well as on top.

Don't overheat your baby. If you leave the baby in the pram or pushchair when you come indoors from outside (perhaps because he is asleep) take the covers off and any heavy outdoor garments.

- A sun canopy or a parasol is useful in summer, and essential when it's very hot. Make sure your baby is out of the direct sun at all times.

- A shopping tray or basket is handy. The ones that fix underneath won't tip your pushchair over when full, if the baby starts wriggling.

- A safety harness to ensure your child is strapped in. This is not necessary for very young babies who always lie down in the pram or pushchair, but it is essential for older babies and toddlers. You will also need one to fasten your child in the high chair.

Sleeping and crying

SLEEPING PATTERNS, AND WHAT TO DO ABOUT CRYING

New babies only ever sleep for a few hours at a time, and it's normal for them to need feeding in the night. It helps if you can get back to sleep as soon as you can after you have fed your baby. Don't switch on the light, or change your baby's nappy unless you have to. Take your baby into bed to feed so you can relax and your baby stays warm.

Your baby can sleep in a cot or crib next to you for the first months. Later, if you prefer, the cot can be in another room. Some parents sleep better if their baby is in a separate room quite early on. Do what suits you, but if

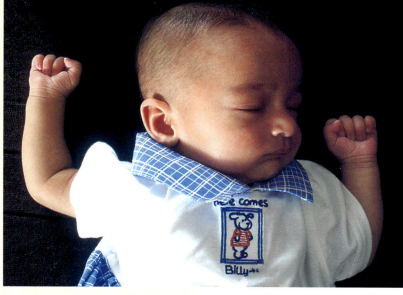

the baby is close to you, you will hear as she wakes, and can start feeding before she gets upset. Don't worry that you are starting 'bad habits'. It's normal all over the world (and throughout history) for mothers and babies to sleep close to each other.

In daytime, young babies can nap in a pram or carry-cot anywhere in the house. As they get older, they are more likely to be disturbed by noise and activity, and you may find your baby sleeps better in a bedroom.

Babies' sleeping habits change as they grow, but these habits vary widely at all ages. It's not realistic to expect your baby to sleep several times a day, waking only for feeds and happy, smiling, socialising ... a few babies may behave like this, but most don't.

All babies have days when they seem to want to sleep more or are more wakeful than usual. Many babies need more attention in the afternoons and evenings, when they may be irritable and demanding.

A baby who seems unusually sleepy may be unwell.

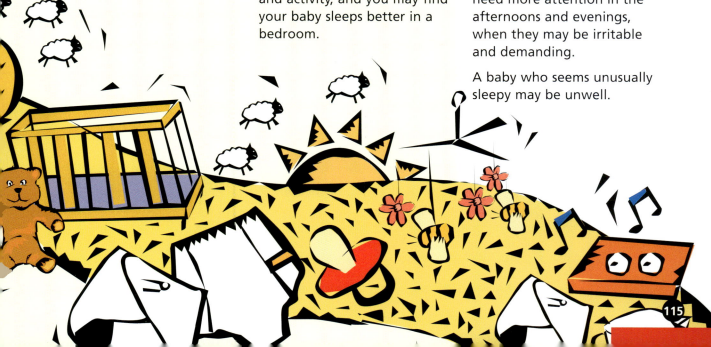

Cot death — reducing the risk

Cot death, or sudden unexpected death in infancy, claims less than 50 infants a year in Scotland. It's rare, and we don't yet know what causes it. We do know, however, that there are ways of reducing the risks. Here's how.

- Place your baby on her back to sleep.

- Don't smoke during pregnancy or afterwards. If it's not possible to have a smoke-free home, **never** smoke where the baby sleeps. Carers should also not smoke near a baby.

- Place your baby's feet at the foot of the cot, to prevent wriggling down under the blankets and overheating. Make the bed up so that the covers reach no higher than the baby's shoulders.

- Don't allow your baby to become too hot — a good guide is to have the temperature of the sleeping place no warmer than is comfortable for a lightly clothed adult.

- Don't use a duvet on your baby's cot, and don't wrap the baby up too warmly. To check if your baby is too hot, feel if she is sweating or feel if the tummy is hot. Don't worry if hands or feet are cold, that is normal. Babies who are unwell need fewer, not more bed clothes.

- Seek medical advice if your baby seems ill with a raised temperature, breathing difficulties or seems less responsive than usual.

In the light of recent research, the Department of Health has issued the following advice (updated June 2004).

- The safest place for your baby to sleep is in a cot in your room for the first six months. While it's lovely to have your baby with you for a cuddle or a feed, it's safest to put your baby back in their cot before you go to sleep. There is a link between sharing a bed all night and cot death if you or your partner:

  - are smokers (no matter where or when you smoke)
  - have recently drunk any alcohol
  - have taken medication or drugs that make you sleep more heavily
  - are very tired.

- Never sleep with your baby on a sofa or armchair.

Older babies and toddlers

Many older babies and toddlers wake in the night. About half of all one year-olds wake up at least once most nights. Many grow out of this by themselves. You may or may not regard it as a problem — for some families, it's just a fact of family life, neither good or bad. They cope, perhaps by sharing a bed with the baby all night, or after she wakes.

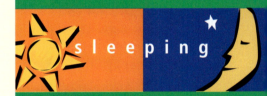

If it worries you, or you find you are tired and irritable after a broken night, you can try to teach your baby to sleep through (see page opposite).

Children who find it hard to settle to sleep may be helped by a calming evening routine before bedtime. Perhaps a bath followed by a quiet half hour with books or songs. At bedtime, make sure your child is happy and comfortable, and don't prolong the 'goodnight'. Leave a light on if this helps, and if she cries, follow the pattern of soothing and calming without fuss suggested in the **Q&A** opposite.

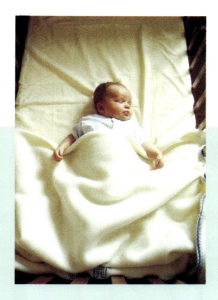

Daytime naps

Most older babies and toddlers sleep at some point in the day until the age of two or three. Some are bad-tempered and irritable if they don't have a nap.

You can encourage a nap at the same time each day (more or less) if you want to. Day nurseries find the children get used to expecting this after a short time, though some babies and toddlers may need help to calm and settle.

Families with toddlers who have trouble settling at night, and in getting back to sleep after waking, are often encouraged to build a nap into the daytime routine. This teaches the child that falling asleep is easy, and prevents the irritable tiredness that makes settling problems worse.

Some children manage perfectly well without a daytime sleep. It's not essential, and may not be what you or your child want.

Q. Can I teach my baby to sleep through?

A. The wakeful baby may not wake up any more often than any other baby. The problem lies in getting back to sleep after waking.

You can change this, though, *if you want to*, after your baby is around seven or eight months old.

When your baby cries, just do what is necessary to settle her — then leave. Eventually, your baby will go back to sleep. Don't leave the baby crying for longer than a few minutes. Soothe and calm by talking, cuddling, stroking her back — but leave it at that. Repeat this again and again and again. Don't do anything else — no playing, feeding, and so on. In this way, you can teach your baby to fall back to sleep by herself. This programme may take a week or a fortnight to work, but if you stick at it, it works. You can discuss it with your health visitor.

Q. When should my toddler use a bed instead of a cot?

A. Most babies are in a cot until the age of about two or three, when they simply get too big. If your child learns to climb out of the cot before this time, you may need to make the move sooner, to prevent accidents. If you need the cot for a new baby, leave a few weeks between moving your toddler out of the cot, and the new baby in.

Crying

Some babies cry a lot more than others, and we don't really know why. They are difficult to soothe and seem miserable a lot of the time, although they may be healthy and developing well. If you are worried about your baby's crying, ask your doctor to check her over to reassure you that all is well. If no cause is found, you may just have to accept that this is the way your baby is. It isn't your fault, and you're not doing anything wrong. In time your baby will become happier and more settled.

Some people believe that persistent crying is caused by colic, due to bubbles of wind. If you think this is the cause, you can try medication from your doctor or the chemist, or traditional remedies like gripe water. Follow the instructions on the bottle and give your chosen remedy three or four days to work.

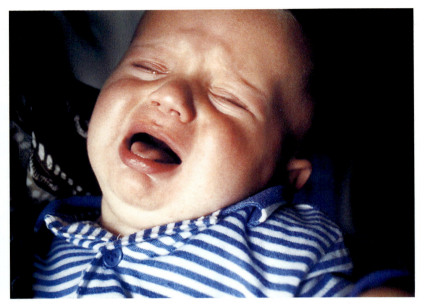

Constant crying in a baby is exhausting and demoralising for you. If you get upset yourself, you may need to put your baby down somewhere safe, or let someone else hold her, and leave the room.

It's worth working through a list of possible 'soothers' to help both of you.

● Rocking, patting or gently rubbing your baby's back or tummy.

● Try a baby soother tape, available from large music stores.

● A baby sling, to carry your baby close to you much of the day.

● More frequent breastfeeds — some babies would like 24-hour access if given the chance!

● A warm bath.

Don't worry about 'spoiling' your baby — you are just offering much needed comfort.

For older babies (from three months) a door bouncer can be hung from the top of a doorway. It has an up-and-down movement which some crying babies love.

If you want to try any complementary therapies, talk to your midwife or health visitor about them.

Always see your doctor if you are concerned about your baby's crying, to check there is no underlying health problem. Get help and support. It can be extremely stressful trying to cope with a baby who seems unhappy. Some parents can become very upset and angry themselves when this goes on for a long time. Don't ever shake your baby — it can be very dangerous. See Further help for support groups.

YOUR DEVELOPING CHILD AT-A-GLANCE PROGRESS

These stages are guidelines only. If you are concerned about your child's development, have a word with your doctor or health visitor.

MONTHS 1–2	MONTHS 3–4	MONTHS 5–6	MONTHS 7–8	MONTHS 9–10
Holds head up for short period of time Legs less bent when lying on tummy	Kicks vigorously Keeps head up with little or no support Lifts head up when placed on tummy with forearms on floor Back straighter when held in sitting position From 4 months—starts to take own weight when held in standing position	Sits with support Rolls front to back Lying on tummy raises up on palms	Sits unaided Might shuffle along floor	Might pull self into standing position May walk anytime between 8–20 months Can reach out for a toy when sitting without falling over
Turns head and eyes towards light	Follows moving object with eyes Watches own hands	Grasps small objects Constantly looks around	Loves watching people	Uses index finger to poke small objects
Responds to your voice	Turns head to follow sound Makes noises	'Speaks' tunefully to self and others	Accurately locates sounds Babbles and responds with noises Shows happiness and annoyance	Understands some phrases
Begins to smile more	Laughs and chuckles when played with	Puts things in mouth Plays with feet Holds arms to be lifted	Drinks out of cup with spout Can start to eat finger foods (from 6 months)	Copies some sounds and actions (eg coughing, waving) Stiffens in annoyance
More awake and alert				
	Less frequent feeds	From 4 months — moving on from milk only		
	May sleep through the night			
Immunisations (from 2 months)		Teething starts at about 6 months		

More over page

119

YOUR DEVELOPING CHILD AT-A-GLANCE PROGRESS

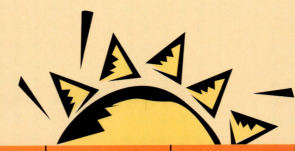

MONTHS 11–12	MONTHS 13–18	MONTHS 19–24	YEARS 2–2½	YEARS 2½–3
Walks around furniture and may start walking alone	Walks and can carry larger objects Climbs up and down stairs with adult help	Runs and falls down less often	Runs, climbs and squats easily	Walks up and down stairs Can catch a large ball
Recognises people from some distance Points	May start to show preference for right or left hand Scribbles with crayon	Better manipulative skills	Copies simple shapes with pencil and paper	Distinguishes between some colours Draws recognisable forms
Understands more complex phrases Responds to own name	Holds 'conversations' Tries to repeat words May have between 6–20 words	Uses simple sentences and asks simple questions Responds to simple instructions	Asks questions Tells you stories	Communicates clearly
Shows affection Finds toys hidden in front of his eyes	Feeds self Restless and curious Enjoys putting things in and out of containers	Pretend play Uses own name	Plays with other children	Makes up games Washes hands and face Counts to 10 if taught
	MMR immunisation		Toilet training	

120

Months 1–2

EVERY DAY IS DIFFERENT

In the first days after birth, some babies are alert but most babies sleep when they're not feeding. Feeds tend to be short, as the baby often falls asleep or becomes drowsy after a few minutes sucking.

Babies like this will probably be more wakeful after a few days, and will spend longer over feeds. (Some aren't like this — they are alert from the very beginning.) Each day can be different. Your baby feeds and sleeps at unpredictable times without much of a pattern.

As the weeks go on, if things go well, you will become more confident and find it easier to keep your baby contented. Feeding will be easier.

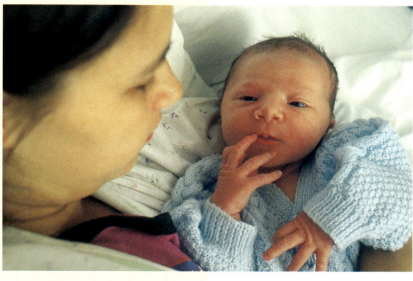

YOUR BABY LEARNS A LOT IN THE FIRST TWO MONTHS

- Hold your baby out in your arms, on his or her tummy, your hands under the chest. By a month your baby will hold his head up in line with the body for a short time.

- From five or six weeks your baby 'coos' in response to your voice and attention.

- From the same age your baby begins to smile more often, and stops whimpering to listen to your voice, and turn his head towards it.

- If you lie your baby tummy-down, you'll notice that the limbs get less 'tucked in'. A newborn bends the knees and draws them up in a 'frog-like' pose, buttocks humped up. By two months this is much less marked. The legs are bent but less drawn up and the bottom is not as high. (Remember, don't let your baby sleep in this position. Babies should lie on their backs to sleep — see page 116.)

- By two months, your baby will be awake and alert more, and need less frequent feeds. Feeds may take less time, too.

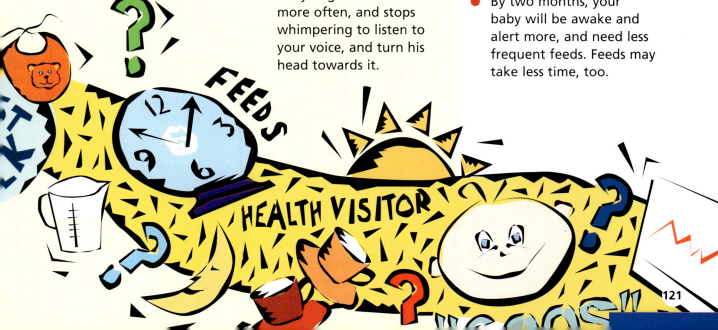

GETTING TO KNOW YOUR HEALTH VISITOR

Your health visitor is a nurse with special training in the health needs, and promotion of good health among families with children under five.

You may meet your health visitor when you are pregnant. About 11 days after the birth of your baby, the health visitor will probably visit you and your baby at home. Your health visitor will tell you about the baby clinic, and when you can bring your baby for immunisations, and talk about progress.

The health visitor's role is to support you, your family and your baby. You can discuss sleep, feeding, weaning, and the baby's development, as well as any aspects of your own feelings and health.

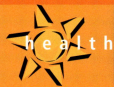 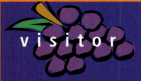

Your child will be offered the first progress check, or routine developmental assessment, at around six to eight weeks. Others are at seven to eight months, at about two, and then shortly before school entry. Your doctor or health visitor will carry them out, either at the clinic or at your home.

At the first check, the assessor will do some basic physical checks, ask you about your baby's progress and answer any questions you may have.

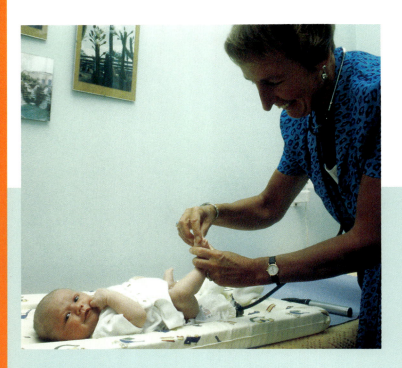

THE CHILD HEALTH CLINIC

You and your baby will be invited to visit the child health clinic. At the clinic, you can ask questions, have your baby's health and growth assessed, and get information about baby care.

Weighing is one useful way of assessing your baby's health. Parents often like to know how their baby is growing. Your health visitor will show you your baby's line on the 'centile' chart. For example, a baby on the 50th centile is average. He weighs more than 49 babies of that age out of every 100, and less than another 49 babies of that age out of every 100. There is also a centile chart for length. Weight is only one part of your baby's progress, though. The baby's overall health and development are most important (see also the development chart on pages 119–120).

There may be a doctor at the child health clinic, to give a medical opinion when needed.

Months 3–4

YOUR BABY IS CHANGING

Babies of this age are getting stronger and chubbier. Their faces, arms and legs 'fill out' and any family resemblances become clearer than before.

You can tell your baby recognises you and maybe one or two other familiar faces. The baby knows what to expect from certain routines now, and shows excitement — for instance, when you are getting a bath ready.

Feeds take less and less time, apart from in the evening when it's still quite common for your baby to need a lot of cuddling, feeding and other attention before settling. You can think about beginning an evening routine around now. This may mean you have some time to yourself once your baby is asleep.

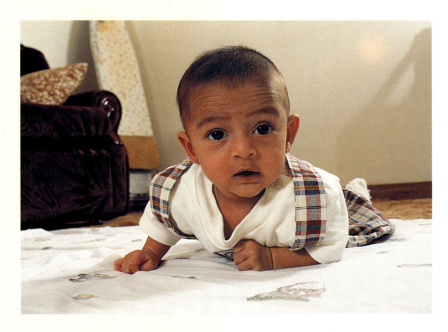

A few babies now sleep through the night.

Here's what else your baby is likely to do:

- when placed in a sitting position, keeps the head up, with little or no lag. (Must be supported.)

- when held in a sitting position, the back is straighter than before

- when placed on tummy, lifts his head and uses forearms to support the upper body

- be a vigorous kicker, and loves lying on his back, having a spot of 'exercise'. May grab a foot and bring it up to the face for a closer look

- when you ring a little bell behind the baby, moving it around, his head will turn to follow the sound

- the baby likes a standing position on your lap, and by four months may be starting to take a little of his own weight.

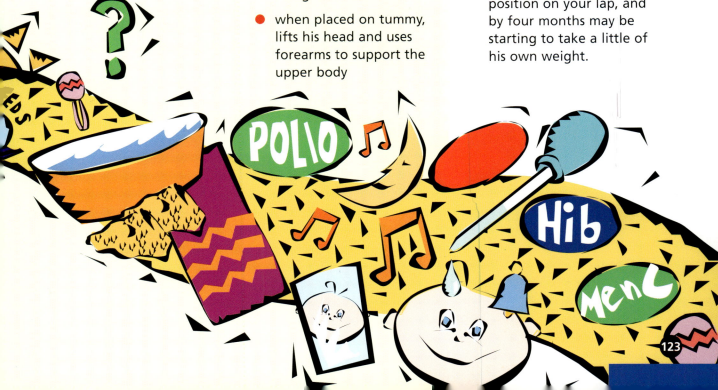

PLAYING WITH YOUR BABY

This is the time when babies start to discover just how sociable they can be, and they begin to realise they have an effect on other people. If they respond to your attention, they'll get more of it!

Watch your baby's reactions when you play, and how she can now move the 'game' along. Here are some play ideas:

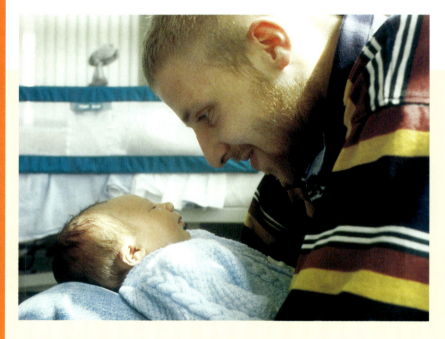

- put a rattle or a small toy in the baby's hands. From about three months babies can hold things, and over the next few weeks hand and eye coordination develops. Your baby will then hold the toy where she can study it for a short time

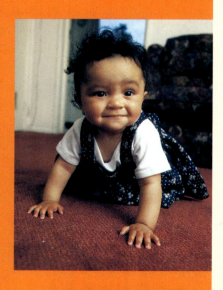

- take your baby to the mirror and look at and talk to 'the baby' in it. Your baby won't realise who this is, but will recognise you. She's not puzzled, though. She just accepts everything

- play with different noises, and see her delight. Try to discover which ones she likes best

- put out your tongue and make funny faces. Your baby may even try to copy you!

- sing songs and hear your baby join in with his own noises

- dangle an object in front of your baby's face. Watch his eyes track its movement from side-to-side and up and down

- sometimes, babies play on their own, studying the shapes their fingers and hands make, moving their blanket to make shadows on the wall, pressing their palms together, waving their hands in front of their face.

Above all, talk to your baby. He can't understand your words, but can hear the shapes and sounds of human speech. Your baby is learning all the time about expression, mood and communication.

Further information on your baby's immunisations can be found in *A Guide to Immunisation for Babies up to 15 Months of Age.*

YOUR BABY'S IMMUNISATIONS

You will be offered three sets of immunisations for your baby in the early months — at two, three and four months of age. Please see the table below for details.

During 2004 a new vaccine called **DTaP/IPV/Hib** was introduced to protect your baby against diphtheria, tetanus, pertussis (whooping cough), polio and Hib meningitis. In this new vaccine the polio part is given in the same injection, unlike the previous vaccine which was given by mouth.

Your baby will also receive the MenC vaccine, which offers protection against meningitis and septicaemia cause by meningococcal group C bacteria, at the same time as DTaP/IPV/Hib.

The **MMR vaccine** protects your child against measles, mumps and rubella. Rubella is also known as German measles. This is given in one injection, usually around 13 months of age. Your local GP surgery will have a copy of the leaflet *MMR: Your questions answered*, and *The MMR Discussion Pack* which helps parents review the facts and discuss any concerns with a health professional.

There are very few reasons why babies cannot be immunised. However, if your baby is clearly unwell or running a temperature, tell your doctor, health visitor or practice nurse and your appointment can be rearranged.

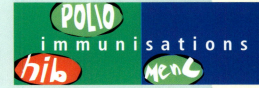

If you have any questions about immunisation, speak to your doctor, health visitor or practice nurse.

Immunisation Timetable		
When to immunise	What vaccine is given	How it is given
Two, three and four months old	Diphtheria, tetanus, pertussis (whooping cough) polio and Hib (DTaP/IPV/Hib)	One injection
	MenC	One injection
Around 13 months old	Measles, mumps and rubella (MMR)	One injection
Three years four months to five years old	Diphtheria, tetanus, pertussis and polio (dTaP/IPV or DTaP/IPV)	One injection
	Measles, mumps and rubella (MMR)	One injection
10 to 14 years old (or sometimes shortly after birth)	BCG (against tuberculosis)	Skin test, then, if needed, one injection
13 to 18 years old	Tetanus, diphtheria and polio (Td/IPV)	One injection

Months 5–6

YOUR BABY'S PROGRESS

Your baby may be sleeping through the night at this age, though it is still normal to wake up. Most babies don't actually need a feed when they wake. They may get one, though, as it's certainly a useful way of comforting crying babies and soothing them back to sleep.

Your baby now chuckles and laughs readily when you play together. He shows anger by squeaking or screaming suddenly rather than tearful crying. The baby now enjoys watching other babies and children. He tries to attract other people's attention by making a noise or waving arms and hands excitedly.

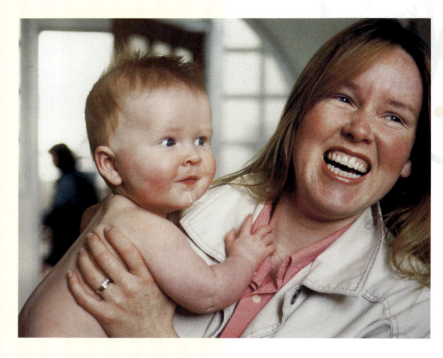

Here are some progress signs during these two months:

- lying on her back, your baby can raise a foot to her face, to play with it, or to suck her toes

- can sit up with support in the pram or on the sofa with cushions around (don't leave her alone like this). Some babies can already sit up by themselves for a few moments

- holds her arms out to be lifted up

- rolls over from front to back and sometimes from back to front

- lying on her tummy, raises her head well up and straightens her arms, with the palms of her hands on the surface

- loves bouncing in a standing position on your lap, or on the floor, while helped to stay 'standing', and takes all her weight on her legs

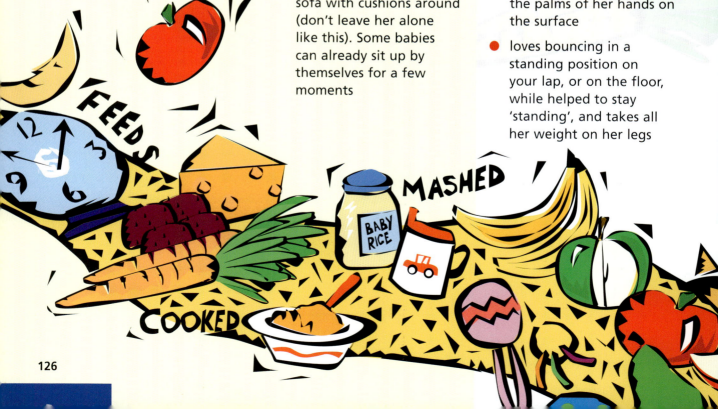

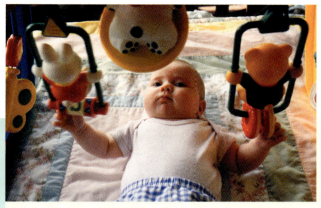

- can grasp small toys and objects put in front of her, usually using both hands

- if she drops something from the pram she watches it fall. If it disappears, she forgets it quickly, not realising you can look for things and find them again! To her, it doesn't exist any more

- uses her mouth to explore everything

- knows that if she shakes a rattle it makes a noise

- cries or 'crumples' her face if you talk to her crossly

- can pass small objects from hand to hand

- adores rough and tumble play.

MOVING ON FROM MILK ONLY

The word 'weaning' means changing your baby's diet to include foods and drinks other than breast milk or infant formula milk. Sometimes, this is called moving on to 'solids' or 'solid foods' — though at first what you offer your baby may not actually be solid in texture. Babies still taking much of their nourishment from breast or formula are said to be 'on mixed feeding' or on a 'mixed diet'.

It has been agreed, both worldwide and in the UK, that breast milk provides all the nourishment that most babies need until they are about six months old. Some babies may need other foods before this, but these should not be introduced before four months at the very earliest.

By the time your baby is **about six months old** she:

- can begin to chew as well as suck

- can swallow food from a spoon, using the tongue to move the food from the front to the back of the mouth

- is curious about other tastes and textures

- is reaching a sociable age and can appreciate the fun of joining in with what other people are doing

- is developing eye-hand coordination which means they start trying to pick things up and put them in their mouth.

First non-milk foods

Very first foods

You don't have to buy anything special. Here are foods suitable for your baby while weaning:

- cooked potato or sweet potato

- baby rice

- cooked swede or turnip

- cooked carrot

- cooked dessert pear, peeled

- cooked dessert apple, peeled

- banana.

Don't cook with or add any salt, seasoning or sugar.

Mash, sieve or puree to get rid of lumps.

Offer small quantities at first, and only one or two new tastes every few days. A couple of teaspoons at a time may be all your baby will want at first. He may even turn his head away at that. Healthy babies know their own appetites, and forcing the issue only makes mealtimes a source of frustration and anxiety.

Don't offer foods containing gluten, egg or cow's milk at this stage (see page 136).

Offering solids

Once a day is fine at first — before, after or even during your baby's milk feed — do what suits you. Later, you can all begin to share mealtimes. Some babies take three months or more to build up to breakfast, lunch and tea; others get there very quickly. **You can offer a cup for drinking from around five to six months.**

A suggested day's eating — at about six months

7 am — breast milk.

8 am — breakfast of baby rice.

11 am — drink of plain boiled, cooled water.

12 midday — midday lunch of mashed potato and dhal. Small slice of dessert apple. Breast milk or formula milk.

3 pm — breast milk or formula milk plus a slice or two of banana.

5 pm — tea of cubed, cooked carrot and peas, mashed potato and chicken, breast milk/formula milk or plain boiled, cooled water.

7 pm — bedtime breastfeed/formula feed.

These times are approximate only. You may find that each day is different for you and your baby.

Don't avoid lumps and chewy foods for too long. Some babies get so used to smooth textures that they won't eat anything with lumps until well into toddlerhood. Mashing with a fork is sufficient for most foods, even for a baby starting solid food.

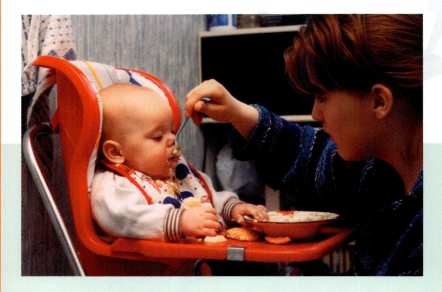

LEAD IN DRINKING WATER

If you live in a house with lead pipes or a lead-lined storage cistern, or if your house has a lead pipe leading to it, the water coming into your house may have a high level of lead in it. Although lead in water is no longer a major health problem in Scotland, it is still important to ensure that lead levels in drinking water are kept as low as possible to prevent any effects on the intellectual development of children.

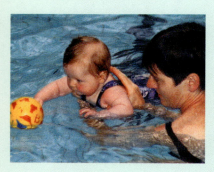

The human body absorbs lead easily from drinking water. Bottle-fed babies, because their intake of water through formula milk is so high, absorb much more than an average adult. And there is evidence that infants retain more lead than adults.

Present levels of exposure to lead in drinking water do not have serious health effects, but can have subtle effects on a child's intellectual development. You will want to ensure your child is not disadvantaged in this way.

You can contact your Environmental Health Department and ask for a sample of your household water to be analysed for the lead levels. (This is a service you may have to pay for.) Water authorities recommend you replace lead pipework and plumbing. Meanwhile, always take water for you or your child from the mains-fed cold tap (usually the tap at your kitchen sink), and always run the mains tap first thing every morning for a minute or two to clear any water in the system that may have been in contact with lead overnight.

For information on vitamin drops for your baby, see page 138.

Months 7–8

TEETHING

By now, most babies have one or two teeth, usually the bottom two incisors (front) teeth. It's quite normal for your baby to have no teeth at all until a year old, and some babies don't get any until after this. You can clean your baby's teeth twice daily with a soft baby toothbrush and a tiny amount of fluoride toothpaste. For more information about caring for your baby's teeth, see page 141.

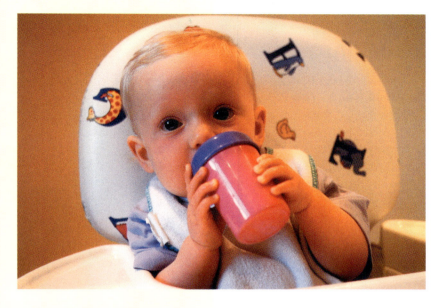

Does teething cause pain?

There's no real explanation for the way that teething babies can sometimes seem distressed when a tooth is coming through. Why should a perfectly normal happening like teething cause the baby any pain?

For some babies, a day or so's restlessness can ease once a tooth comes through. Babies dribble more, too, at this time, and this can cause soreness on the cheeks and the chin.

Sugarfree teething gels rubbed on the gums seem to help some babies.

If your baby seems listless and unhappy, don't think these are just teething troubles. It may be illness. Contact your doctor.

SITTING UP, TAKING NOTICE

At this age your baby:

- can sit up unaided for several minutes

- may be able to move along the floor by sliding or shuffling. Some babies are skilled rollers! A few can crawl

- can hold a cup with a spout and drink

- can locate sounds quite accurately, turning the head to the correct side to listen to your voice or to the sound of a toy

- can babble and respond to you with noises.

WHO IS THIS PERSON?

By now, you and your baby have really got to know each other. You can see a real little person who can 'tell' you what he likes and dislikes. You may be able to tell if your baby will be placid and easy-going later on, or excitable and needing constant entertainment and fun — quiet and shy, or outgoing and noisy! Like all human beings, your baby may behave differently in some situations and with different people.

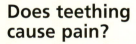

129

YOUR BABY AND OTHER PEOPLE

It's very common for babies to show some degree of wariness or even anxiety towards strangers at around this age. Babies often turn away and bury their face in your shoulder if someone strange tries to talk to them.

Your baby may respond to someone else's approaches, but only when you are there.

For some babies this lasts just a short time; for others, it continues and may get worse. Your baby may hate it if you go out of the room, and you may have to call out to show you are still around. Your baby doesn't yet know that when you are out of sight, you will be coming back.

Most babies have other special people in their lives, and they can link certain actions and items with them. Perhaps your baby knows Grandma's house, and recognises it with excitement as you go up the path. The sound of someone's familiar voice may make him laugh delightedly, knowing who is coming.

Routines are important at this age, and your baby may not like any change in the pattern of the day. If you go away on holiday, your baby may not feel happy about sleeping in a different cot or room. If nap times are changed, he may be grumpy and irritable.

At around seven to eight months your child's hearing and sight will be checked. The child may be given small bricks and you'll be asked about his communication skills. Don't be anxious if your child doesn't 'perform' well. If there is any cause for concern, the assessments can be repeated. You'll be asked about your own observations and experience of what your child can and can't do. These, too, are an important and accurate guide to your child's development.

EATING

Finger foods

Gradually introduce finger foods once your baby has become accustomed to soft/mashed/pureed foods. Finger foods are foods your baby can pick up and eat himself, without any help from you. Some babies never really enjoy solids until they're at this stage — usually from about six months, depending on when you started weaning — and they seem to prefer managing themselves instead of being spoon fed. Some babies move through the pureed food stage quickly, particularly if they have been introduced to solids later (nearer to six months).

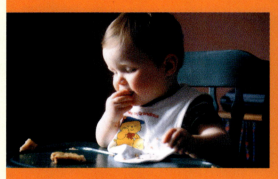

Cut or slice the foods up into a shape your baby can hold easily, to chew, gnaw or suck at. Good finger foods are:

- slices of bread, toast, pitta, nan or chappati
- slices of eating apple, pear
- sticks of carrot, celery, cucumber
- tiny sandwiches with grated cheese, cottage cheese, pure fruit spreads, mashed banana
- savoury cheese biscuits (those without salt)
- fingers of cheese on toast or pizza
- cubes of cheese
- cooked pasta shapes — bow shapes or chunky macaroni are easy to pick up
- cooked vegetables.

Note: always stay with your baby when he is feeding, in case of choking.

Don't offer finger foods containing gluten, egg or cow's milk until at least six months of age.

For more information on eating in the second six months see page 136.

SAFETY AND YOUR CHILD

Being careful about safety begins from your baby's earliest days.

In a car

The baby needs to ride in a rear-facing baby seat until he can sit unaided for a long time. These seats can be used wherever there is a lap/shoulder seat belt. BUT you must NEVER place them on the front seat if the car has a passenger airbag.

At home

Many parents are taken by surprise when their baby learns to roll. You turn your back for a few moments, and the baby has moved! Never leave your baby or toddler unattended on a raised surface at any age. He may roll off and get hurt.

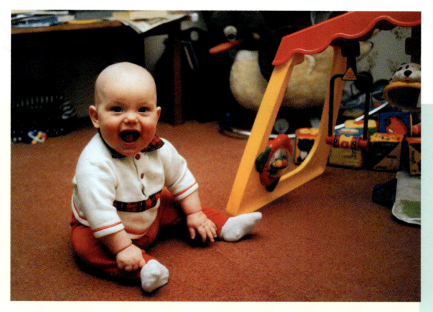

Look out for:

- trailing flexes from electrical equipment
- open electrical sockets — buy plastic socket covers to block the holes from tiny fingers or block off access to sockets with heavy furniture

- pet paraphernalia — cat litter trays, food bowls, baskets
- hanging tablecloths
- small objects, such as an older child's toys, left on the floor
- hot drinks. **Don't** drink them with a baby on your lap.

Take action

- Fit a smoke alarm preferably on every floor of your home, if you haven't already, and check it is working regularly.
- Know how you and the family can leave your house quickly in an emergency such as a fire.
- Fit fire-guards to open fires or stoves.
- Keep a well-stocked first-aid kit in the kitchen and the bathroom.

- Keep vital numbers (doctor, hospital, partner's work number and so on) by the phone for quick reference by anyone in an emergency.
- Place safety gates at the top and bottom of stairs. Use one across the doorway at times you want your baby to keep out of a room, such as the kitchen. You can still see and 'talk' to each other.
- Don't place objects on the stairs — you could easily trip when carrying your baby, or learner climbers can trip, or harm themselves on the objects.
- Fit safety catches on cupboard doors, low drawers, fridge, freezer — anywhere you store dangerous or messy objects.

> **Dangers increase when your baby's crawling, cruising round the furniture or walking.**

131

- Keep poisons (including medicines and tablets, bleach, cleaning materials, weedkillers) out of reach and locked away.

- Always place hot liquids, pans, tea and coffee pots and pans well out of reach.

- Turn saucepan handles to the back of the stove and use the back rings whenever possible.

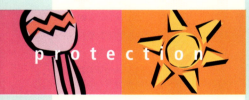

protection

- Apply safety film or fit safety glass on any low level glass surfaces, including doors and tables.

- Fit a guard over the controls of the video and TV.

- Prevent doors slamming shut on your child's fingers by using a door stop. Or tie a cloth across the front and back handles, which stops the door shutting completely.

NEVER leave your child in the bath alone, or alone near any water indoors or out — even a few inches in a bucket is dangerous.

When children are able to talk, teach them their full name. Some two-year-olds can manage to say their address, and even their phone number. This can be vital if ever your child gets separated from you in a shopping centre or other busy place.

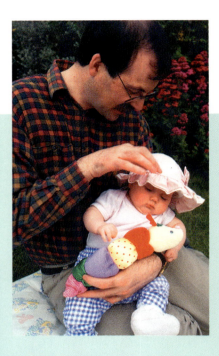

Sun safety

Always protect babies and toddlers from sunshine. Babies under six months should be kept out of direct sunlight altogether. Keep your child in the shade whenever possible, and use a sunhat or sunshade on the pram or pushchair. If your child is outside on a sunny day, on the beach or in the garden, and crawling or walking, it can be hard to provide shade at all times. Use a child sun-screen cream with a high protection factor (at least 25). Put a T-shirt and hat on your child, and stay indoors in the middle of the day during a British heatwave (or every day if you are holidaying somewhere very hot). Your child will also need more to drink in the heat.

Your health visitor may know of loan schemes which allow you to borrow safety equipment, or hire it for a small charge.

Months 9–10

MOVING AROUND

Most babies can crawl by 10 months, and some can 'cruise' round the furniture. Most can also pull themselves to a standing position with furniture of the right height — but they can't get to the floor again without falling down with a bump.

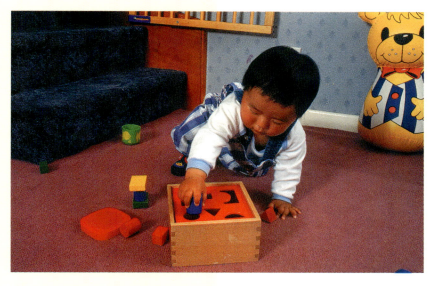

WHAT ELSE ARE THEY DOING?

Your baby may still be 'clingy'. Babies who haven't gone through this stage may do so now. In somewhere strange, or with new people, they want to stay on your lap, or very near you.

Here are some other skills babies develop at this age. They:

- are quite stable when sitting, and can turn and stretch out to grasp a toy without always toppling over

- can use the index finger to poke at a small object. If they see a hole they try to stick their fingers in it. (Protect electric sockets with special covers.)

- bring their fingers and thumbs together in a pincer movement to pick up something small

- feed themselves quite well with 'finger foods', but cannot yet use a spoon

- babble with recognisable sounds, like 'mamama' and 'dadada', and can imitate some sounds that you make

- love copying funny noises like raspberries and kissing sounds

- can refuse to cooperate with you, stiffening the body if you want to dress them, and protesting noisily at the same time

- understand phrases like 'no', 'bye bye' and 'dinner'

- watch while you hide a toy under a cloth, and know the toy's still there, triumphantly removing the cloth

- copy your actions to produce an effect. For example, ring a bell, show it to them, give it to them, and they wave it to make the same noise.

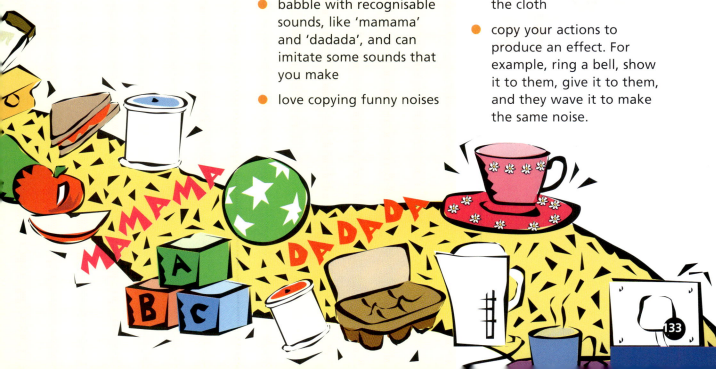

PLAYING WITH YOUR BABY

By now, babies are very interested in toys that have some sound, and movement. They can use their fingers and hands to open little doors or to push things along. Show your baby what to do, and enjoyment and curiosity will make her copy you.

Babies love examining and handling different objects, and anything easy to hold is fascinating. Check that things are safe, and can't be swallowed. Your baby will enjoy handing you items, and taking them from you as you hand them back.

Put together a busy box for you both to play with together. Talk about the things you're playing with, describe them and say what your baby's doing with them — 'Yes, you're touching that and it's all rough on that side, and this side's smooth ...' Here are some suggestions for your box — you can keep changing the items so there's always something new to study.

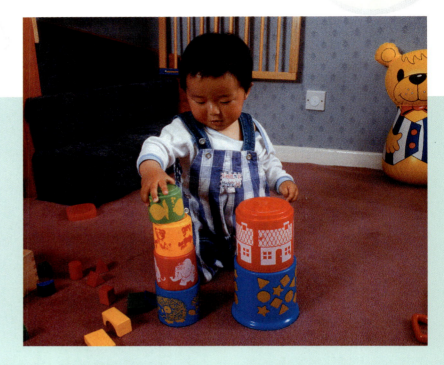

- Empty cotton reels.
- Small plastic bottles (throw tops away).
- Scraps of different-textured fabrics.
- Spoons.
- Doll's cup and saucer.
- Wooden bricks.
- Egg cartons.
- Ball.
- Crackly paper.

Babies enjoy **finger games** and **hand games**, like *Round and Round the Garden* and *This Little Piggy*. They learn to look forward to the tickly bit at the end. Your baby may take your hand and make you do it again when you've stopped. Clapping games help your baby's coordination

skills. Help your baby to make music, by singing and providing banging and rattling toys to join in with.

Play 'peep-bo' and 'boo', and watch the delight as the baby learns that although you're hiding, you're still there.

Watch how your baby starts games. For example, babies learn that dropping a toy from a high chair means you pick it up ... and if they do it again, you pick it up again, and again, and again!

Your health visitor can help you with some ideas for games if you don't know any, or if you have forgotten them.

Months 11–12

YOUR NEARLY ONE YEAR-OLD

By the end of the first year your baby is showing the first signs of wanting to make decisions, and may get annoyed if you don't agree.

In many ways babies love to cooperate with you. They hold their arms out for their jacket, for example. They often wave 'bye bye' when asked, and try to brush their hair if you give them a hairbrush or comb. They will hand you objects if you ask and offer your hand, and may be able to point to familiar things. But if you say 'Where's Mummy's nose?' they are just as likely to point to their own nose.

Here are some other abilities which show you how far your baby has come in this one year.

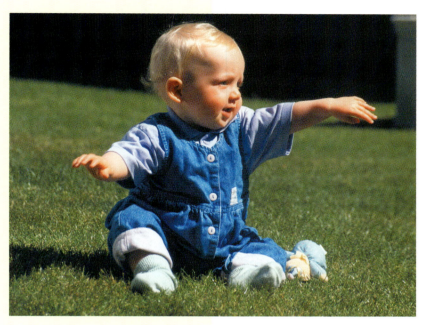

- They can point at an object, so that you'll comment on it, such as, 'Yes, that's a light', 'Yes, you can see a car'. We know they do this to get a response, as babies don't do it when they are alone.

- They may walk at any time from 8 months to 20 months, and some babies may try to climb the stairs (fit stair gates to prevent accidents).

- Non-walkers may bottom shuffle or crawl very quickly, or 'bear walk' using arms and legs extended.

- They can recognise people they know from some distance.

- They know their own name and turn in response to it.

- They understand more complex phrases such as 'Where is the cup?' and 'Do you want a drink?'

- They show affection with cuddles and kisses.

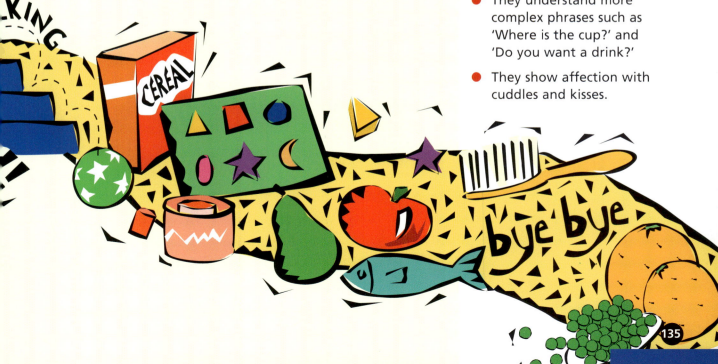

FAMILY MEALS — EATING IN THE SECOND SIX MONTHS

As well as breast and/or formula feeds, most babies have a breakfast, a lunch and a tea, and small snacks in between, by the time they are nine months, and many reach that stage earlier. There is a greater variety of food in the diet now, and most foods are suitable for your baby after six months. By this stage (or a little older, depending on when you first introduced non-milk foods) you can start introducing foods that you have been delaying until now.

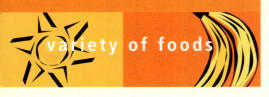

variety of foods

New foods include:

- cereals containing gluten. Gluten is present in wheat, and in foods containing wheat, including bread and many breakfast cereals, and most flour products (pasta)

- well-cooked egg yolks from six months and then the white at about eight months

- hard cheese (grated, melted or cubed).

Limit fried foods, and anything very spicy. Don't add salt or sugar to your baby's food.

Avoid nuts. Children who are believed to be sensitive to peanuts should continue to avoid such foods until they are at least three years old, and advice should be taken on obtaining a medical diagnosis. It is also advised that children under five years should not be given whole peanuts because of the risk of choking.

You can use ordinary cow's milk in small amounts in cooking from about six months, but until the baby is at least a year old, the best milk for him to drink is breast milk or formula. Tea is not advised for a baby or toddler — it prevents the absorption of iron.

It's normal for your baby's appetite to vary from day to day, and some babies seem to start eating rather less towards the end of the first year. That's fine, as long as your baby is healthy and happy, and continues to grow, even if the weight gain is a lot slower now.

Ready-prepared baby foods

Most babies will eat ready-prepared, bought baby foods. They're normally made without added salt or artificial additives. They are a useful stand-by and also convenient to use.

However, your baby doesn't need to have any bought baby foods. Preparing your own food may take a little longer, but it's definitely worth making sure your baby has regular chances to experience the variety of textures and tastes in homemade food. Some babies who have a lot of baby foods may not want to try the 'real' stuff, and some actually gag on the lumps and

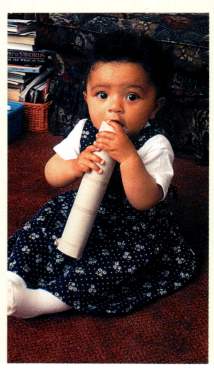

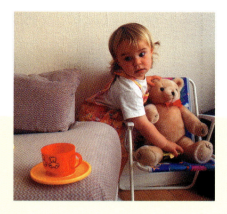

'bits' in it. It may take a lot of patience to get them to enjoy family meals.

The nutritional content of ready-prepared foods is worth considering. Added sugars make baby foods, desserts in particular, very sweet indeed. Many baby foods have a high water content and this means they also need to use starchy thickeners. While these may do no harm, they are low in food value, and don't represent good value for money either.

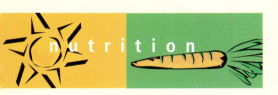

Read the labels on baby foods, to avoid the highly sweetened varieties, and the ones with a high water and starch content. Thickeners are labelled as vegetable gum, gelatine, modified starch and different types of flour. You may also see the term 'maltodextrin'. This is a starch-based bulking agent of little nutritional value.

As with pre-prepared foods for adults, the main ingredient is listed first on the label. You'll find you pay more for better quality baby foods, with a low water and starch content.

Q. When should my baby use a cup?

A. Start introducing a cup at any time around five to six months. Your baby will need help at first.

Q. When should my baby stop breastfeeding?

A. It's up to you. Continue to breastfeed for as long as you and your baby choose. The World Health Organization recommends that babies are breastfed for at least the first year but preferably well into the second year and beyond. Worldwide, many mothers breastfeed for more than a year. Any amount of breastfeeding has valuable health advantages, and breast milk is always a healthy drink, whatever your baby's age. See *Breastfeeding: Getting Off to a Good Start*, available from your health visitor or local health promotion department.

Q. And what about bottles?

A. Bottles are different. A baby still taking several bottles of milk a day could well be filling up with milk, and not getting vital nutrients from other foods. Aim to phase out your baby's bottles by the age of a year or so, apart from perhaps a bedtime one (don't let your baby sleep with it in her mouth). If your baby is very keen on bottles, do this gradually, offering a cup with meals, and taking a cup when you go out visiting.

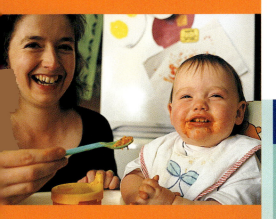

A suggested day's eating — at about 11 months

7 am — breast milk/ formula milk.

8 am — breakfast of scrambled egg, toast, breast milk/formula milk or plain boiled, cooled water.

10 am — breast milk/ formula milk.

12 midday — lunch of lamb and mashed carrot and potato, satsuma, breast milk/formula milk or plain boiled, cooled water.

3 pm — breast milk/ formula milk, breadstick.

5 pm — tea of yoghurt, cracker, portion of mashed banana, breast milk or formula milk.

7pm — bedtime breastfeed/formula feed.

These times are approximate only. You may find that each day is different for you and your baby.

q u e s t i o n s   a n s w e r e d

Q. Is a vegetarian diet enough for a baby?

A. Yes. Your baby does not need meat or fish to stay healthy. Vegetarian babies can get the necessary protein and other nutrients from other parts of their diet — pulses, eggs, milk, grains and cereals.

A vegan diet — which excludes animal products like eggs and milk — can be healthy for a baby, too, but there is a risk that the diet may not include enough of certain nutrients. It is a good idea to speak to a dietitian if you are thinking of weaning your baby onto a vegan diet. Speak to your health visitor or GP to arrange this. For more information you can write to the address on page 155.

For more information about healthy eating, see page 13.

What about vitamin drops?

Your health visitor or GP will give you advice on infant vitamin supplements. They are usually given to babies as liquid drops. The current official advice is that bottle-fed babies over six months who take less than 600 ml (about a pint) of formula each day may need vitamin supplements. From six months, babies receiving breast milk as their main drink need to be given supplementary Vitamin D, and in some cases Vitamin A.

Babies and children over a year on a varied diet may not need supplements.

Months 13–18

BECOMING A TODDLER

Most children learn to walk during these months, though a few may be 'bottom shuffling' or 'bear walking' so well that they don't try to walk properly until later. Children can now walk and carry one or two large toys at the same time without losing their balance. They can walk up and down stairs with adult help. By the end of this period they can climb into a full-size chair, or squat on the floor to play or to pick something up.

Children can control their hands and fingers, and build a small tower of three bricks, if you show them what to do. They may now show a preference for the left or the right hand — watch which one they use when you offer crayons or pencils.

At mealtimes, they use a spoon fairly well. They are much less likely to explore every object they pick up with the mouth. They love to

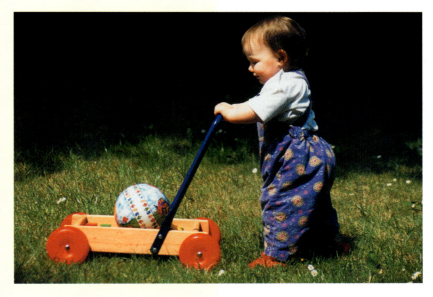

explore — knobs, cupboards and drawers fascinate them. They want to see behind doors. This is the start of a period that can be quite physically exhausting for you — you seem to be running round after your child all day, and needing eyes in the back of your head!

Understanding and communication skills grow a great deal in this time. Children can:

- put things in and out of a container, and play with a simple shape sorter after practice

- use anything between 6 and 20 words in 'conversation'

- repeat words or try to do so when asked

- try to sing and to join in with songs

- learn 'party tricks' such as telling you what the dog says, or what the cow says

- talk to themselves, while playing. You may hear your child say 'No' when about to do something she knows you won't approve of.

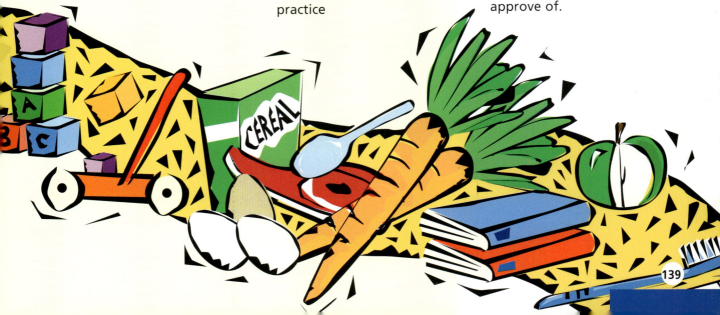

Books and your baby

You can introduce books to your baby from the very first weeks. Start by enrolling your baby in your local library, and by buying some books she can look at on your lap.

Books for your baby can be any size and shape. Babies seem to prefer small, strong, sturdy books, with pages that can be turned easily.

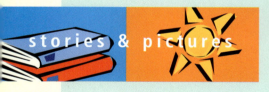

From about six months, your baby learns to anticipate, and to pick up clues that something familiar is about to happen. Babies enjoy books where they know what's going to be on the next page. They can learn from this. A book where a baby gets dressed, with a new garment put on on each page, is a 'story' that's just right for a baby from about nine months.

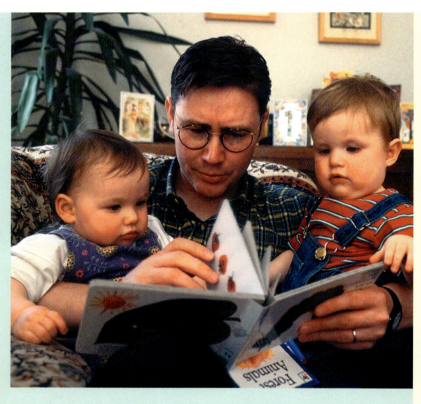

When you show and talk about these books to your baby, relate the pictures to her own life and routine. When the book baby has socks on, for example, show your baby her socks. When you see a face, point to the nose, eyes and mouth and so on, and then point out your baby's, and your own, nose and eyes and mouth.

Have some paper books you don't mind your baby messing up — old mail order catalogues are wonderful for babies — they love the sections with the babies in. Make your own scrap books for your baby to look at, and put in pictures you know are special and relevant. Include a few photos of friends and family, and the baby. If your baby gets excited at dogs, or cats, or cars, have lots of pictures of these.

YOUR CHILD'S TEETH

Start good habits by:

- brushing your baby's teeth as soon as they appear with a baby toothbrush

- using only a tiny amount of ordinary fluoride toothpaste — a smear on top of the brush

- avoiding giving your baby sugary snacks and drinks between meals, and keep high sugar foods to a minimum

- giving water to drink, or if you give fruit juice, dilute it with water (1:10) and only offer at mealtimes. Don't offer sweet drinks in bottles or as a soother before naps or at bedtimes.

- never leaving your baby with a sweet drink in a bottle (or feeder cup) — this can lead quickly to decay of the top front teeth.

Register your baby with a dentist at any time from six months, or when the first tooth comes through and take him along for visit. Arrange regular visits and ask your dentist about fluoride supplements.

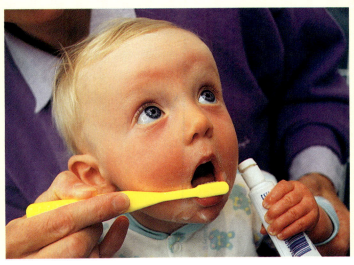

EATING

Iron

Research shows that some babies and toddlers in the UK don't get enough iron in the foods they eat.

This important mineral is essential for health and development. Some children who are short of iron are listless, lacking in energy and have a poor appetite. However, others appear happy and healthy, and the deficiency isn't diagnosed.

Iron is found in red meat, eggs, cereals, pulses, dried fruits and some vegetables. Your baby needs more iron from about six months. Breast milk and infant formula supply some of the iron, but your child needs it from other sources, too.

Make sure your child has enough iron

- In the first year, give your child breast milk or infant formula as a drink, rather than cow's milk (whole pasteurised milk) which is comparatively low in iron.

- Offer at least one serving per day of a food containing iron from the age of six months.

- Serve food containing Vitamin C. Vitamin C helps the body to absorb iron, and is found in fruits and vegetables (raw or lightly cooked to preserve the Vitamin C content).

Don't give your child tea to drink. It reduces the absorption of iron.

Months 19–24

LEAVING BABYHOOD BEHIND

By the end of this period, children can run, and they fall down much less often. They can propel themselves forward (and often backwards as well) on a small trike, but very few children can use the pedals yet. They attempt to kick a large ball, by walking into it and then kicking their feet out.

During this time, climbing and 'acrobatic' skills develop. Children will now use imagination when trying to get something that's out of reach — pulling a chair or a table across to use it as a platform. They can show concentration, and their hands are steady enough to build a tower of six or seven small bricks. Their manipulative skills show — they can turn the pages of a book one at a time, and unwrap a sweet.

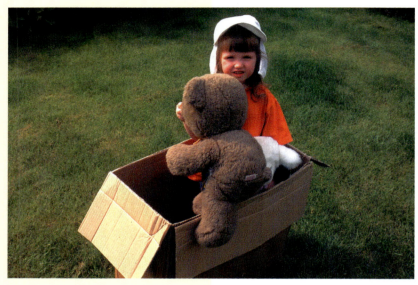

Children enjoy copying people, and by two, they like pretend play with, say, dolls, teddies or cars. They show determination and anger when stopped from doing something they want to do. They may not like sharing toys. They can be very demanding about getting attention. They enjoy the company of other children, but still can't play with them in any meaningful way, and may show aggression towards them. Tantrums and displays of temper are very common.

Your child may show great progress in speaking, talking and listening, and can:

- put two words together, sometimes three or more, to make a simple sentence ('Mummy, Mummy ... go home now?')

- ask questions about the surroundings ('What's that?')

- know her own name and use it

- respond to easy instructions, such as 'Go and get the dog's lead'.

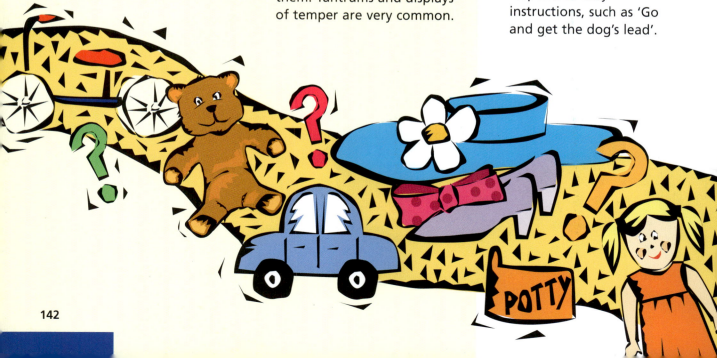

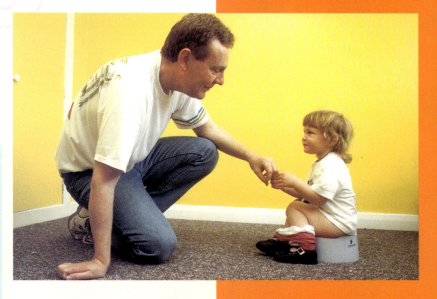

TOILET TRAINING YOUR CHILD

You can start teaching your child about bladder and bowel control at some time around the second birthday, though for some children, this is too soon. Children are usually ready for learning about it when they:

- understand simple commands like 'Put your shoes on the floor'

- go for a couple of hours without a wet nappy

- manage to help you when getting dressed and undressed

- know when they have opened their bowels or bladder.

If your child is at this stage, and you don't have any other major events going on in your family at present (like a house move, a holiday or a very new baby), then you can try training.

Tell your child what you are planning to do, and if you can, show her what other children do. Visit the toilet together, and explain what you are doing in a way she can understand.

Here are some suggestions you can follow.

- If you recognise when your child needs to open her bowels, sit her on the potty. If the child manages to do something, give lots of praise. If not, just be casual about it.

- If you have a couple of hours or more at home with your child, don't put on a nappy. Every so often, see if the child will sit on the potty. You may be able to prolong the time spent there by looking at a book together. Again, if something happens, give praise and encouragement.

- Increase the opportunities to use the potty or the toilet, and offer occasional reminders about it.

It helps if you:

- have a potty downstairs and upstairs, for quick access

- have spare pants and a bag for the wet ones when you go out.

Accidents will happen. Almost all toddlers will wet or soil themselves many times before they are reliably trained. If your child wets or soils several times a day, it may be too soon for training. There is no shame in going back to nappies, and it may be much less stressful. Stay calm when your child has an accident. Simply clean up, and tell your child it doesn't matter.

Disposable trainer pants are sometimes helpful for this in-between stage. They absorb 'the accident' so it doesn't go through to the outer clothing, yet they can be pulled up and down like normal pants for use with the potty or toilet. However, not all parents like them — some feel they are too much like a nappy, and confuse the not-quite-trained child.

For more information about toilet training, see page 145.

2 – 2½ years

YOUR SOCIABLE CHILD

Now your child begins to be more sociable with other children, playing games where she has to take a turn, without protesting or just not understanding.

Your child may be able to manage her clothing when using the potty or toilet, but probably needs help. A few children are dry at night.

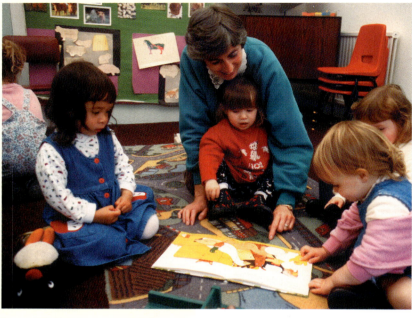

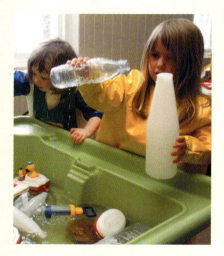

Your child now has confidence in physical skills, and the energy for running around in open, safe spaces. She can copy simple shapes and even letters made up of straight lines (like T or L) with a pencil and paper.

The child can drink from a cup without a lid, and use a fork. Spoon-feeding herself is easy.

Your child's language is more sophisticated, and understandable to people outside the immediate family circle. There will still be difficulty with some sounds, and pronouns (she, me, you, I and so on) may still confuse.

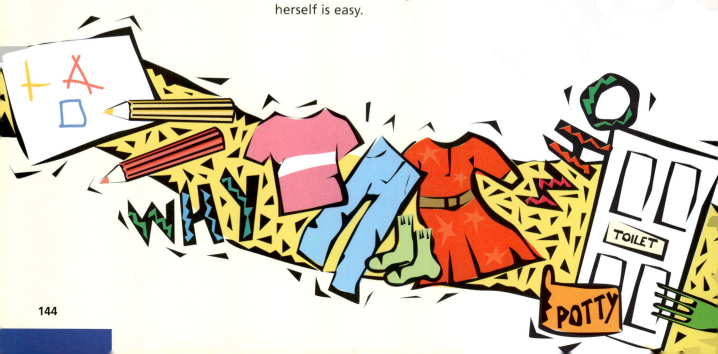

At this stage, children:

- use 200 or more recognisable words and build sentences

- know their full name, and possibly address or town (if you teach this)

- ask questions with words like 'Why' and 'Who'

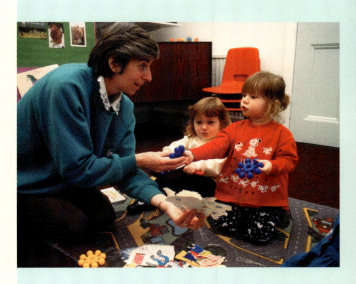

- can fill in the missing word when you read from a familiar story book, or sing a song he knows well

- can tell you of events that have happened and/or are about to happen.

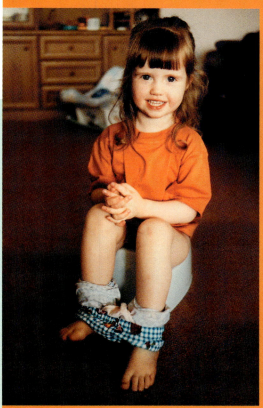

MORE ON TOILET TRAINING

Toddlers of two-and-a-half or so who haven't yet used the potty may be able to skip the potty stage altogether. They may be big enough to get on the toilet with help. A toddler seat can give extra comfort and security at first. It helps if you encourage your child to use a toilet from the start, at least from time to time, to avoid having to take a potty with you everywhere you go.

Before the age of about two-and-a-half, most children are not able to 'hang on' more than a very short time when they want to use the toilet.

2½ – 3 years

YOUR ACTIVE CHILD

By the end of three years, your child is agile, energetic and confident, and moves efficiently. He can walk upstairs and downstairs with alternating feet (when coming downstairs, children usually jump from the bottom step, with two feet together). He can stand on tiptoe and walk in this way, and stand on one foot without wobbling over straight away.

If you throw a large ball, your child can catch it, usually on or between the arms, rather than with the hands. He can ride a trike using the pedals.

Now your child can use a pencil to draw a recognisable human form, with a head, arms and legs, or other features. He begins to know colours. Red and yellow usually come first, and it may take longer to tell blue from green.

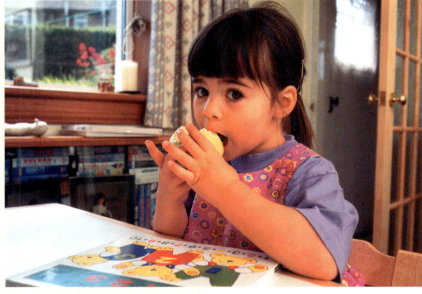

Most children are able to dress and undress themselves, at least partially, if their clothing is simple. They can wash their hands and face, though they may need help with proper drying.

They can start to share, and they join in pretend play with other children, often making up quite elaborate games with playthings.

They can communicate with family and others well and clearly, and enjoy keeping a conversation going.

- They can count to 10 if taught, but don't really understand the concept of numbers beyond two or three.

- They know several nursery rhymes by heart.

- They can tell you how old they are.

- They use pronouns correctly and pronounce more accurately.

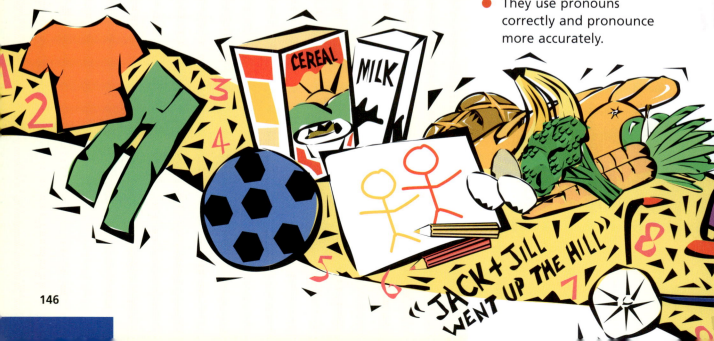

Q. How can I teach my child to be dry at night?

A. Night-time dryness usually comes after daytime dryness. While most children achieve this at about three, it's common for some to be wet at night until five or six or more. Wait until you have a few dry night nappies, and then leave them off, telling your child what you are doing and why. Make it easy for your child to go to the toilet at night. If you decide to take your child to the toilet at night, make sure you wake him. Otherwise you are teaching him to urinate in his sleep, which is exactly what you don't want to happen.

Night-time wetting is not usually considered a problem until the age of about seven, as so many children simply grow out of it.

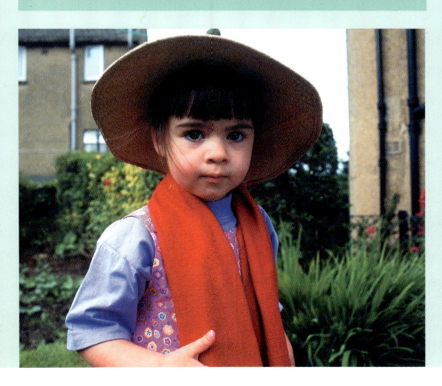

HEALTHY EATING FOR YOUR CHILD

Toddlers need foods from all the different food groups (see page 13), but their need for energy-rich foods is higher than an adult's. Toddlers can't eat a large amount of food at any single meal, they prefer small meals with snacks between them. High fibre foods (eg wholemeal bread, pasta and breakfast cereals) can be very filling but are low in energy. Offer a mixture of ordinary and wholemeal versions of these products.

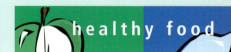

healthy food

A good, healthy diet for your child will include vegetables, fruit, bread, cereals and grains (rice, pasta, breakfast cereals), meat and fish, milk, eggs, dairy products (cheese, fromage frais, yoghurt).

If your child has a good appetite you can introduce semi-skimmed milk from age two.

If your child is vegetarian, pulses (lentils and beans) and soya foods will be needed to replace the meat and fish (otherwise the rest is the same). Keep sweetened and sugary foods to a minimum, and continue to follow the advice on dental health on page 141.

Eating problems

Eating problems are common in the toddler years. There are times when children seem to eat a lot more, or a lot less, than at other times. They may 'go off' foods they've always liked, or develop favourite foods which they used to reject.

This is all very natural — children have likes and dislikes, just as you do. They are developing their independence, and want to make choices. They want to choose what they eat just as they want to make decisions over other things in their daily life.

With some children, their developing preferences can spring from a different source — it's as if they want the familiar and the 'safe', in a world which is still, in part, a bewildering collection of different and unexpected events and activities.

Parents worry that these eating habits can lead to poor nutrition. It's also annoying to have a child whose behaviour at the table is upsetting and who continually says 'No' or who has to be persuaded all the time to eat things.

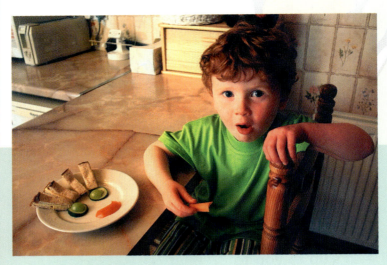

However, making a fuss over your toddler's eating habits risks making her more difficult to handle. Here are some ideas to help:

- offer your child small quantities, cut up into bite-sized pieces

- offer gentle encouragement and praise when she eats

- if food is rejected or only a few mouthfuls eaten, accept the child's 'verdict' and remove the plate

- always have something to eat when your child eats, to make the mealtime a social occasion. This will also help to divert your attention from her plate

- let the child feed herself

- never force feed

- don't make food into a disciplinary issue (like saying 'It's naughty to leave your dinner' or making threats)

- have your child weighed to reassure you about growth

- don't allow filling up on milk between meals

- snacks are fine, but don't give anything too substantial too close to a meal

- if your child asks for something an hour after a rejected dinner, don't make a fuss. Provide something — but don't make snacks generally more appealing than the meal

- don't talk about your child's eating habits in front of her.

Sometimes, problems do get worse, and a child's health suffers as a result. They may not get all the nutrients they require.

A child may not gain weight satisfactorily, or stick to such a limited diet of sweetened foods that teeth are affected.

These effects are rare, but they need to be checked for. Your health visitor or doctor can arrange for a full health check and perhaps a consultation with a dietitian.

Remember, even very young children can be moody — don't worry unduly and remember to seek advice and reassurance from your health visitor.

Illness and what to watch out for

Babies and small children can't tell you when they aren't well — it's up to you to decide whether your child is feeling ill, and how seriously to take it.

Most babies will have some 'off days' in their first year — mild feverishness can bring a few bouts of irritable, restless crying. Occasionally, symptoms are not mild, and you need to get help. Sometimes you're worried about puzzling symptoms, and you need to know from your doctor whether there is anything seriously wrong. Mild illnesses such as coughs or colds are common. They can be worrying for you, so do seek advice if you are concerned. Severe, life-threatening illness is very rare in babies and young children.

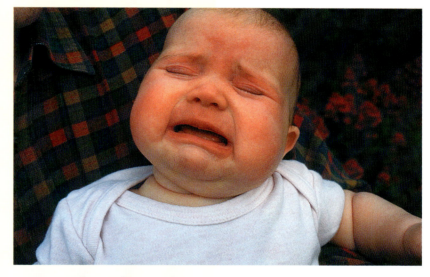

See your doctor (or speak on the phone) if your baby:

- seems listless, or much less alert than usual, or sleeps for an unusually long time

- has continuous vomiting which lasts more than an hour

- has diarrhoea which doesn't clear up in a day

- has a rash which you can't explain by it being a heat rash or a result of clothes rubbing

- has dry nappies

- passes stools which are an unusual colour or texture for him (green stools from time to time are nothing significant, and some baby formulas result in green stools routinely)

- seems feverish and uncomfortably hot (check the chest rather than the forehead — if the skin feels sweaty and hot, the child probably has a temperature)

- has unexplained bruising or bleeding from the ears, mouth, nose, anus or in the stools or the urine.

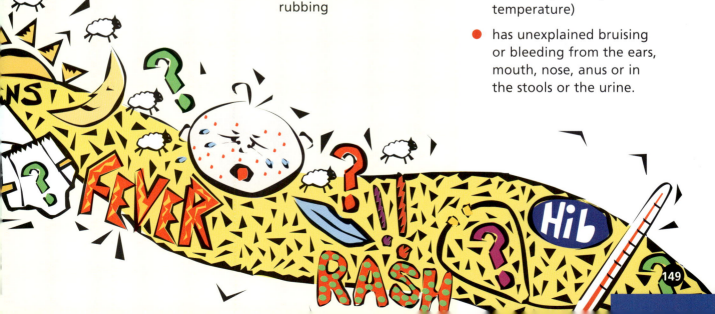

Seek medical help straight away if your baby:

- has a convulsion — continuous twitching or jerking with unfocused, rolling eyes and a lack of response

- has breathing difficulties

- loses consciousness

- becomes blue around or on the lips or the face

- has signs or symptoms of suspected meningitis and septicaemia (see opposite)

- passes blood or redcurrant-jelly-like stools

- seems in obvious pain.

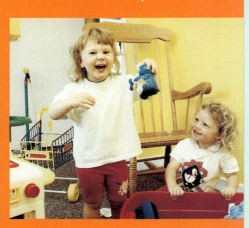

Although babies who scream for a long time are very worrying to parents, babies who are really ill don't cry continuously and loudly. If your baby is making such a noise, he is basically okay, though of course may be in distress or uncomfortable. Constant whimpering and moaning is more likely in a baby who is poorly.

For more information on crying see page 118.

Your doctor may not always prescribe medication for your baby — sometimes it's not appropriate, as your baby doesn't need it.

MENINGITIS AND SEPTICAEMIA — WHAT TO LOOK FOR

Meningitis is an inflammation of the meninges, the protective membranes covering the brain and spinal cord. Different forms are caused by bacteria, and by viruses. Meningitis is rare, but can be a very serious illness. If it's diagnosed and treated early, the majority of children make a full recovery.

Septicaemia — blood poisoning — is caused by the same bacteria which causes most cases of meningitis. It is extremely dangerous.

The Hib vaccine protects against Hib meningitis only, and no other forms. MenC vaccine protects against meningitis and septicaemia caused by meningococcal group C bacteria. There are other causes of meningitis and septicaemia, so it is important to stay alert. If you suspect that your child may have meningitis or septicaemia then get medical help immediately. Acting quickly could save their lives.

Signs and symptoms of meningitis and septicaemia

The early signs and symptoms of meningitis and septicaemia can be difficult to spot because they can be similar to flu. Signs and symptoms include:

- vomiting
- fever
- pain in the back or joints
- bad headache
- stiff neck.

Later signs and symptoms include:

- dislike of light
- a bruise-like rash which doesn't fade under pressure (do the 'Glass Test', see below)
- confusion
- drowsiness leading to coma.

The rash starts as tiny red pinprick spots or marks and later changes to purple blotches, which can look like bruises or blood blisters. The rash can be anywhere, and will not fade when pressed with the side of a glass — the 'Glass Test'.

Signs of meningitis and septicaemia in babies may also include:

- tense or bulging fontanelle (the soft spot on the baby's head)
- blotchy or pale skin
- refusing to feed
- fretfulness or dislike of being handled
- high-pitched moaning cry.

Remember — remain alert to the signs and symptoms of meningitis and septicaemia. It is important to get medical help immediately if you think someone has meningitis or septicaemia. These are dangerous and can develop very quickly. The earlier people are treated, the better the chances are of making a full recovery.

For more information on meningitis and septicaemia, see the Further help section at the back of this book.

TRUST YOUR INSTINCTS. IF YOU THINK YOUR CHILD IS ILL, GET HELP

Further help, information and useful addresses

The following organisations may be able to put you in touch with local sources of help in your area. Those outwith Scotland may have details of Scottish contacts. Call them for assistance and a friendly chat. Many of them provide helpful leaflets on request. Where they exist telephone helpline numbers have been included — you may wish to contact them for helpful advice, counselling or simply for general information.

A very useful service which provides information about where to find help is available locally through your local health education/promotion unit which is listed under 'Health' in your phone book and/or the **NHS Helpline Freephone: 0800 22 44 88** (all calls free of charge; 8am-10pm, 7 days). Your public library is also an invaluable source of information. For further information about any health-related issues, please contact:

NHS Health Scotland Library
The Priory, Canaan Lane
Edinburgh EH10 4SG
Tel: 0845 912 5442
Textphone: 0131 536 5593
email: library.enquiries@hebs.scot.nhs.uk
www.healthscotland.com/library

ABUSE

Children 1st
83 Whitehouse Loan
Edinburgh EH9 1AT
Tel: 0131 446 2300
Fax: 0131 446 2339
email: info@children1st.org.uk
www.children1st.org.uk
Offers practical help to families with children at risk.

ParentLine Scotland
0808 800 2222
Confidential and anonymous telephone helpline run by volunteers for parents/carers.

Scottish Women's Aid
Norton Park
57 Albion Road
Edinburgh EH7 5QY
Tel: 0131 475 2372
Fax: 0131 475 2384
email: info@scottishwomensaid.org.uk
Advice, support and refuge to women who have been abused mentally, physically or sexually, and their children.

ACCIDENT PREVENTION & SAFETY

British Red Cross Society (Scottish Region)
Alexandra House, 204 Bath Street
Glasgow G2 4HL
Tel: 0141 332 9591
Provides a range of caring and first-aid services and courses.

Child Accident Prevention Trust (CAPT)
4th Floor, Clerks Court
18-20 Farringdon Lane
London EC1R 3HA
Tel: 020 7608 3828
Fax: 020 7608 3674
email: safe@capt.org.uk
www.capt.org.uk
Offers help and advice to parents on the prevention of childhood accidents.

The Royal Society for the Prevention of Accidents (RoSPA)
Slateford House, 53 Lanark Road
Edinburgh EH14 1TL
Tel: 0131 455 7457
www.rospa.com
Information and advice on the prevention of accidents of all kinds.

St Andrew's Ambulance Association
St Andrew's House
48 Milton Street, Glasgow G4 0HR
Tel: 0141 332 4031
email: firstaid@staaa.org.uk
www.firstaid.org.uk
Provides training in first-aid and related subjects.

ADOPTION

Scottish Adoption Association
2 Commercial Street, Edinburgh EH6 6JA
Tel: 0131 553 5060
email: info@scottishadoption.org
www.scottishadoption.org.uk
Offers a comprehensive adoption service including advice and counselling to anyone affected by adoption.

ALCOHOL, DRUGS & SMOKING

Alcohol Focus Scotland
2nd Floor, 166 Buchanan Street
Glasgow G1 2LW
Tel: 0141 572 6700
Fax: 0141 333 1606
email: enquiries@alcohol-focus-scotland.org.uk
www.alcohol-focus-scotland.org.uk
Provides free, confidential counselling services for people affected by alcohol problems. Promotes safer, healthier drinking styles, but is not anti-alcohol.

Alcoholics Anonymous (AA)
50 Wellington Street, Glasgow G2 6HJ
Tel: 0141 226 2214
Helpline: 0845 769 7555
Fax: 0141 221 9450
Network of self-help groups where members encourage each other to stop drinking and to stay off drink. Look in the phone book for details of your local group.

ASH Scotland
8 Frederick Street, Edinburgh EH2 2HB
Tel: 0131 225 4725
Fax: 0131 225 4759
email: ashscotland@ashscotland.org.uk
www.ashscotland.org.uk
Information and resources to encourage smokers to quit.

FRANK (National drugs helpline)
0800 77 66 00
www.talktofrank.com
Free 24-hour confidential drug information, advice and counselling service.

Scottish Drugs Forum
Shaftesbury House
5 Waterloo Street, Glasgow G2 6AY
Tel: 0141 221 1175
Fax: 0141 248 6414
email: enquiries@sdf.org.uk
www.sdf.org.uk
Offers information on local treatment and services for drug users, family and friends.

Smokeline
0800 84 84 84
Scottish national helpline for smokers who need advice or help in stopping, or their friends who are encouraging them to stop. Staffed by trained counsellors who can send you a free copy of a helpful guide.

BEHAVIOURAL DIFFICULTIES

Hyperactive Children's Support Group
71 Whyke Lane, Chichester PO19 7PD
Tel: 01243 551313
Fax: 01903 734726
email: hyperactive@hacsg.org.uk
www.hacsg.org.uk
Provides information and ideas to parents and professionals about nutritional/dietary therapies for hyperactive and allergic children.

BREASTFEEDING

Association of Breastfeeding Mothers (ABM)
PO Box 207, Bridgwater, Somerset TA6 7YT
Helpline: 020 7813 1481
email: info@abm.me.uk
www.abm.me.uk
Gives support and information to all women wishing to breastfeed, and counselling around the UK.

The Breastfeeding Network
P.O. Box 11126, Paisley PA2 8YB
Supporterline: 0870 900 8787
email: email@breastfeedingnetwork.org.uk
www.breastfeedingnetwork.org.uk
Offers independent information and support about breastfeeding.

La Leche League (Great Britain)
P.O. Box 29, West Bridgford
Nottingham NG2 7NP
Helpline: 0845 120 2918
email: lllgb@wsds.co.uk
www.laleche.org.uk
Help and information for women wanting to breastfeed their babies and personal counselling to mothers having problems in breastfeeding. Local groups hold friendly, informal discussions on breastfeeding, birth and parenthood.

The National Childbirth Trust (NCT)
Alexandra House, Oldham Terrace
Acton, London W3 6NH
Enq: 0870 444 8707
Breastfeeding: 0870 444 8708
Fax: 020 8992 5929
www.nctpregnancyandbabycare.com
Help and information for women wanting to breastfeed their babies. Breastfeeding counsellors can offer personal support.

CHILDCARE

Daycare Trust
21 St George's Road, London SE1 6ES
Childcare Hotline: 020 7840 3350
Fax: 020 7840 3355
email: info@daycaretrust.org.uk
www.daycaretrust.org.uk
Information and advice on obtaining suitable forms of childcare and on setting up daycare.

National Association of Toy & Leisure Libraries
4 Drum Street, Edinburgh EH17 8QG
Tel: 0131 664 2746
Fax: 0131 664 2753
email: natll.scotland@playmatters.co.uk
www.natll.org.uk
Toy Libraries loan good quality, carefully chosen toys to all families with babies and young children, including those with special needs.

Scottish Childminding Association
Suite 3, 7 Melville Terrace
Stirling FK8 2ND
Tel: 01786 445377
Fax: 01786 449062
email: information@childminding.org
www.childminding.org
Works to promote high quality daycare for children under
eight years and provides help and advice for
childminders and parents.

Scottish Pre-school Play Association
45 Finnieston Street, Glasgow G3 8JU
Tel: 0141 221 4148
email: info@sppa.org.uk
www.sppa.org.uk
Organisation for playgroups, mother-and-toddler groups, and
under-five groups in Scotland.

Working Families
1-3 Berry Street, London EC1V 0AA
Tel: 020 7253 7243
Fax: 020 7253 6253
email: office@workingfamilies.org.uk
www.workingfamilies.org.uk
Helps children, working parents and carers and their
employers find a better balance between responsibilities at
home and at work.

DISABILITY & ILLNESS (GENERAL SUPPORT)

Action for Sick Children
172 Leith Walk
Edinburgh EH6 5EA
Tel: 0131 553 6553
Supports sick children and their families. Offers
information about going to hospital designed for
children and for parents. Hospital playboxes available
for borrowing by playgroups.

**Association of Parents of Vaccine
Damaged Children**
21 Saughton Mains Gardens
Edinburgh EH11 3QG
Tel: 0131 443 9287
Concerned with obtaining adequate compensation for
children damaged by vaccination; also offers support to
families.

Contact A Family Scotland
Norton Park, 57 Albion Road
Edinburgh EH7 5QY
Tel: 0131 475 2608
Fax: 0131 475 2609
email: scotland@cafamily.org.uk
www.cafamily.org.uk
Encourages mutual support between families caring for
children with any type of disability or special need.

Disability Information Trust
Nuffield Orthopaedic Centre
Oxford OX3 7LD
Tel: 07092 746081
email: news@abilityonline.org.uk
www.abilityonline.org.uk
Assesses and tests equipment for people with
disabilities.

Disability Scotland
Princes House, 5 Shandwick Place
Edinburgh EH2 4RG
Tel: 0131 229 8632
Fax: 0131 229 5168
Textphone: 0131 229 8632
email: enquiries@disabilityscotland.org.uk
Information and advice on all aspects of disability: access and
mobility, equipment, community care and daily living
problems.

ENABLE
6th Floor, 7 Buchanan Street
Glasgow G1 3HL
Tel: 0141 226 4541
Fax: 0141 204 4398
email: enable@enable.org.uk
www.enable.org.uk
Promotes the rights and needs of people with learning
disabilities and their families. Can offer information, advice
and practical help.

Family Fund Trust
P.O. Box 50, York YO1 9ZX
Tel: 01904 621115
Government-funded Trust whose purpose is to ease
the stress on families who care for severely disabled
children under 16 by providing grants and information related
to the care of the child.

Genetic Interest Group (GIG)
Unit 4D, Leroy House
436 Essex Road, LONDON N1 3QP
Tel: 020 7704 3141
Fax: 020 7359 1447
email: mail@gig.org.uk
www.gig.org.uk
Information service for people with or at risk of genetic
conditions.

DISABILITY & ILLNESS (SPECIALISED SUPPORT)

Advice Service Capability Scotland (ASCS)
11 Ellersly Road, Edinburgh EH12 6HY
Tel: 0131 313 5510
Fax: 0131 346 1681
email: ascs@capability-scotland.org.uk
www.capability-scotland.org.uk
Offers advice, support and information to parents of children
with cerebral palsy.

AFASIC Unlocking Speech and Language
2nd Floor
50-52 Great Sutton Street, London EC1V 0DJ
Helpline: 0845 3 55 55 77
Tel (admin): 020 7490 9410
Fax: 020 7251 2834
email: info@afasic.org.uk
www.afasic.org.uk
Provides advice and information on speech and
language difficulties amongst children.

Anaphylaxis Campaign
PO Box 275
Farnborough, Hants GU14 6SX
Tel: 01252 373793
Helpline: 01252 542029
Fax: 01252 377140
email: info@anaphylaxis.org.uk
www.anaphylaxis.org.uk
Campaigns to help anyone who suffers from potentially fatal
allergy. Provides help to sufferers and aims to raise awareness
within government, industry and the general public.

**Association for Children with
Heart Disorders**
104 Comiston Road, Edinburgh EH10 5QL
Tel: 0131 447 2711
Provides support to children and young adults with
heart disorders, and their families.

Asthma UK Scotland
2A North Charlotte Street, Edinburgh EH2 4HR
Tel: 0131 226 2544
Helpline: 0845 701 0203
Fax: 0131 226 2401
email: enquiries@asthmas.org.uk
www.asthma.org.uk
Information and support for people with asthma and
their families.

Child Growth Foundation
2 Mayfield Avenue
Chiswick, London W4 1PW
Tel: 020 8994 7625/020 8995 0257
Fax: 020 8995 9075
www.heightmatters.org.uk
Support group for parents of children with growth
disorders, and parents concerned about their child's growth.

**Children Living with Inherited Metabolic
Diseases (CLIMB)**
Climb Building
176 Nantwich Road, Crewe CW2 6BG
Tel: 0800 652 3181
Fax: 0870 7700 327
www.climb.org.uk
Makes grants and allowances available for the
purposes of medical treatment and care of children
with metabolic diseases. Puts parents in contact with others
in similar circumstances.

Cleft Lip and Palate Association (CLAPA)
CLAPA Head Office
1st Floor
Green Man Tower
332b Goswell Road, London EC1V 7LQ
Tel: 020 7833 4883
Fax: 020 7883 5999
email: info@clapa.com
www.clapa.com
Offers support to parents of children with cleft lip and/or
palate. Offers a specialist service to those seeking help in
feeding babies with clefts.

The Coeliac Society
P.O. Box 220, High Wycombe
Buckinghamshire HP11 2HY
Tel: 01494 437278
www. coeliac.co.uk
Advice and information for those with the coeliac
condition or dermatitis herpetiformis.

Craighalbert Centre
The Scottish Centre for Children with Motor
Impairments
1 Craighalbert Way, Cumbernauld G68 0LS
Tel: 01236 456100
Fax: 01236 736889
email: sccmi@craighalbert.org.uk
www.craighalbert.org.uk
Scottish national centre which offers a system of
'conductive education' which aims to teach the cerebral
palsied child all aspects of daily life, develop learning ability
and prepare the child for school.

Cystic Fibrosis (CF) Trust
11 London Road, Bromley, Kent BR1 1BY
Tel: 020 8464 7211
Fax: 020 8313 0472
email: enquiries@cftrust.org.uk
www: cftrust.org.uk
Funds medical and scientific research aimed at understanding,
treating and curing cystic fibrosis. Aims to ensure that people
with the disease receive the best care and support in all
aspects of their lives.

Diabetes UK Scotland
Savoy House, 140 Sauchiehall Street
Glasgow G2 3DH
Tel: 0141 332 2700
Fax: 0141 332 4880
email: scotland@diabetes.org.uk
www.diabetes.org.uk/scotland
Provides practical help and information on living with
diabetes.

Down's Syndrome Scotland
158-160 Balgreen Road, Edinburgh EH11 3AU
Tel: 0131 313 4225
email: info@dsscotland.org.uk
www.dsscotland.org.uk
Information, advice, counselling and support for parents of
children with Down's syndrome.

Eczema Scotland
84 West Main Street
Broxburn, West Lothian EH52 5LQ
Tel: 01506 852 033
Information, advice and support for people with eczema and
their families.

Epilepsy Association of Scotland
National Headquarters
48 Govan Road, Glasgow G51 1JL
Tel: 0141 427 4911
Helpline: 0808 800 2200
Fax: 0141 419 1709
email: enquiries@epilepsyscotland.org.uk
www.epilepsyscotland.org.uk
Charitable organisation working for people with epilepsy,
their families, carers and the professionals looking after them.

Group B Strep Support
P.O. Box 203, Haywards Heath
West Sussex RH16 1GF
Tel: 01444 416176
email: info@gbss.org.uk
www.gbss.org.uk
Provides information for pregnant women,
pregnant women who carry the bacteria, parents
of infected children and health care professionals.

The Haemophilia Society
Chesterfield House
385 Euston Road
London NW1 3AU
Tel: 020 7380 0600
Helpline: 0800 018 6068
Fax: 020 7387 8220
email: info@haemophilia.org.uk
www.haemophilia.org.uk
Represents the needs and interests of people with, or affected by, haemophilia.

Jennifer Trust for Spinal Muscular
Atrophy (SMA)
Elta House
Birmingham Road
Stratford Upon Avon CV37 0AQ
Tel: 0870 774 3651
Fax: 0870 774 3652
email: jennifer@jtsma.org.uk
www.jtsma.org.uk
For those affected by any form of SMA. Can link families and help to provide equipment.

MENCAP, the Learning Disability Charity
Mencap National Centre
123 Golden Lane
London EC1Y 0RT
Tel: 020 7454 0454
email: information@mencap.org
www.mencap.org
Works with children and adults with a learning disability and their families and carers to improve their lives and opportunities.

Meningitis Association of Scotland
9 Edwin Street
Glasgow G51 1ND
Tel: 0141 427 6698/0141 556 4211
Fax: 0141 427 6698
www.meningitis-scotland.co.uk
Free information and support to those suffering from meningitis or who are disabled as a result.

Meningitis Research Foundation
133 Gilmore Place
Edinburgh EH3 9PP
Tel: 0131 228 3322
Helpline: 080 8800 3344
Fax: 0131 221 0300
www.meningitis.org
Offers counselling for parents whose children have died from meningitis and gives support to people with loved ones in hospital or at home. (See also Meningitis Trust, below.)

Meningitis Trust
19 Hillfoot
Houston PA6 7NR
Tel/Fax: 0845 120 4885
Helpline: 0845 6000 800
email: support@meningitis-trust.org.uk
www.meningitis-trust.org.uk
Free information and support to those suffering from meningitis or who are disabled as a result.

Muscular Dystrophy Campaign
7-11 Prescott Place
London SW4 6BS
Tel: 020 7720 8055
Fax: 020 7498 0670
email: info@muscular-dystrophy.org
www.muscular-dystrophy.org
Offers practical help and emotional support to sufferers and their families, runs an information and education service for the medical professions, social services and the public.

National Autistic Society Scotland
Central Chambers
1st Floor
109 Hope
Street Glasgow G2 6LL
Tel: 0141 221 8090
Fax: 0141 221 8118
www.nas.org.uk
Parent support group which runs an advisory and information service.

National Deaf Children's Society Scotland
293-295 Central Chambers
93 Hope Street
Glasgow G2 6LD
Tel: 0141 248 2429/0141 248 4457
Fax: 0141 248 2597
email: veronica@ndcs.org.uk
www.ndcs.org.uk
Information and advice service on all issues relating to childhood deafness. Offers the expertise of specialist advisors in the fields of education, health, benefits and technology.

National Society for Phenylketonuria (NSPKU)
P.O. Box 26642
London N14 4ZF
Tel: 0845 603 9136
Fax: 0870 122 1864
email: info@nspku.org
www.nspku.org
Self-help organisation offering information and support to families affected by the disorder.

Reach (Association for Children with Hand or Arm Deficiency)
PO Box 54
Helston
Cornwall TR13 8WD
Tel: 0845 1306 225
Fax: 0845 1300 262
email: reach@reach.org.uk
www.reach.org.uk
Aims to promote the relief of children with upper limb deficiencies by encouraging mutual aid and support between their families.

RNIB Scotland
Dunedin House
25 Ravelston Terrace
Edinburgh EH4 3TP
Tel: 0131 311 8500
Fax: 0131 311 8529
Information, services and advice for blind people. Look Scotland (0131 313 5711) provides information to parents on services relevant to children with visual impairment.

Scope
PO Box 833
Milton Keynes MK12 5NY
Cerebral Palsy Helpline: 0808 800 3333
email: cphelpline@scope.org.uk
www.scope.org.uk
Provides a range of services for people with cerebral palsy and their families/carers.

Scottish Society for Autism
Hilton House, Alloa Business Park
Whins Road Alloa FK10 3SA
Tel: 01259 720044
Fax: 01259 720051
email: autism@autism-in-scotland.org.uk
www.autism-in-scotland.org.uk
Provides a range of services in care, support and education for people with autism, their families and carers.

Scottish Spina Bifida Association
190 Queensferry Road
Edinburgh EH4 2BW
Tel: 0131 332 0743
Helpline: 08459 111112
Fax: 0131 343 3651
email: mail@ssba.org.uk
Web: ourworld.compuserve.com/
homepages/SSBAHQ
Information, advice, counselling, support and financial help for parents.

SENSE Scotland (National Deaf-Blind and Rubella Association)
45 Finnieston Street
Glasgow G3 8JU
Tel: 0141 564 2444
Fax: 0141 564 2443
email: info@sensescotland.org.uk
www.sensescotland.org.uk
Information, advice and support for families of deaf-blind and rubella handicapped children.

Sickle Cell Society
54 Station Road
London NW10 4UA
Tel: 020 8961 7795
Fax: 020 8961 8346
email: info@sicklecellsociety.org
www.sicklecellsociety.org
Information, advice and counselling on sickle cell disease and traits.

Society for Mucopolysaccharide
Diseases (MPS)
46 Woodside Road
Amersham HP6 6AJ
Tel: 01494 434156
Fax: 01494 434252
email: mps@mpssociety.co.uk
www.mpssociety.co.uk
Acts as a parent support group; brings about more public awareness of MPS diseases; raises funds for research.

Tay Sachs Screening Programme
R26 Research Centre
Royal Manchester Children's Hospital
Pendlebury
Salford M27 4HA
Tel: 0161 794 4696
Screening, information, counselling and practical support to families with present or past history of fatal genetic disorders.

UK Thalassaemia Society
19 The Broadway
Southgate Circus
London N14 6PH
Tel: 020 8882 0011
Fax: 020 8882 8618
email: office@ukts.org
www.ukts.org
Education, information, research and counselling offered to sufferers and carriers. Publicity available in many languages.

FAMILY PLANNING

Caledonia Youth
5 Castle Terrace
Edinburgh EH1 2DP
Tel: 0131 229 3596
Fax: 0131 221 1486
email: information@caledoniayouth.org
Offers free and confidential sexual health services for all young people up to and including the age of 24 years. Help and advice on cervical screening, pregnancy testing, abortion referral, counselling for sexual and emotional problems.

Family Planning Association Scotland
Unit 10
Firhill Business Centre
76 Firhill Road
Glasgow G20 7BA
Helpline: 0141 576 5088
Fax: 0141 948 1172
www.fpa.org.uk
Aims to promote sexual, emotional and reproductive health, together with planned parenthood, by providing information, publicity, education and training.

GENERAL SUPPORT

Caesarean Support Network
55 Cooil Drive
Douglas
Isle of Man IM2 2HF
Tel: 01624 661269 (evenings only)
Provides support and advice on all matters relating to Caesarean delivery, whether recent or in the past.

Couple Counselling Scotland
18 York Place
Edinburgh EH1 3EP
Tel: 0131 558 9669
Fax: 0131 556 6596
email: enquiries@couplecounselling.org
www.couplecounselling.org
Counselling service for couples with relationship difficulties, irrespective of race, religion, marital status or sexual orientation.

Institute for Complementary Medicine
P.O. Box 194, London SE16 1QZ
Tel: 020 7237 5165
Fax: 020 7237 5175
email: icm@icmedicine.co.uk
www.icmedicine.co.uk
Charity providing information on complementary medicine and referrals to qualified practitioners or helpful organisations.

Life
Life House
Newbold Terrace, Leamington Spa CV32 4EA
Tel: 01926 421587
Fax: 01926 336497
email: info@lifeuk.org
www.lifeuk.org
Campaigns for the repeal of the 1967 Abortion Act. Offers pregnancy and post-abortion counselling, and accommodation for women and their babies.

The Infertility Network
Charter House
43 St Leonards Road
Bexhill-on-sea, East Sussex TN40 1JA
Tel: 08701 188088
Fax: 01424 731858
email: admin@infertilitynetwork.uk.com
www.infertilitynetwork.com
Helps couples coping with problems of infertility and childlessness.

The Samaritans
Admin office
The Upper Mill, Kingston Road
Ewell, Surrey KT17 2AF
Helpline: 08457 90 90 90
Tel: 020 8394 8300
Fax: 020 8394 8301
email: admin@samaritans.org.uk
www.samaritans.org.uk

Scotland Patients' Association
Gartincaber
West Plean, Stirling FK7 8BA
Tel: 01786 818008
email: SCOTL1@AOL.COM
www.scotlandpatientsassociation.org.uk
Provides advocacy and information to raise awareness of health matters and issues relating to the delivery of services. Deals confidentially with complaints and queries about health services. Can offer medical and legal advice, and an interpreter service.

Shelter Scotland
Head Office, 4th Floor Scotiabank House
6 South Charlotte Street
Edinburgh EH2 4AW
Tel: 0131 473 7170
Fax: 0131 473 7199
email: shelterscot@shelter.org.uk
www.shelter.org.uk
Works to relieve poverty and distress among homeless people and campaigns for provision of housing to meet need; runs regional housing aid offices and charity shops.

Women's Health
52 Featherstone Street, London EC1Y 8RT
Helpline: 0845 125 5254
Fax: 020 7250 4152
email: health@womenshealthlondon.org.uk
www.womenshealthlondon.org.uk
Information on a wide range of women's health issues. Provides a phone and postal enquiry service, reference library and database to help put women in touch with individuals or groups for self-help and support.

HIV & AIDS

National Aids Trust
New City Cloisters
196 Old Street
London EC1V 9FR
Tel: 020 7814 6767
Fax 020 7216 0111
email: info@nat.org.uk
www.nat.org.uk
Aims to promote a wider understanding of HIV and AIDS; develop and support efforts to prevent the spread of HIV; and improve the quality of life of people affected by HIV and AIDS.

Positive Voice
37-39 Montrose Terrace
Edinburgh EH7 5DJ
Tel: 0131 652 0754 (office)
        0131 477 2580 (volunteers)
Fax: 0131 661 9100
email: enquiries@positive-voice.org.uk
www.positive-voice.org.uk
Offers support, advice and counselling to those who are affected by HIV and AIDS their families, partners and friends.

Positively Women
347-349 City Road
London EC1V 1LR
Tel: 020 7713 0222
Fax: 020 7713 1020
email: poswomen@dircon.co.uk
www.positivelywomen.org.uk
Support agency for women living with HIV/AIDS and their families.

Waverley Care Solas
2/4 Abbeymount
Edinburgh EH8 8EJ
Tel: 0131 661 0982
Fax: 0131 652 1780
email: solas@waverleycare.org
www.waverleycare.org
Supporting people in Scotland living with HIV. Respite unit, information and support centre, buddy programme and women's weekly support group.

LOSS & BEREAVEMENT

The Compassionate Friends
53 North Street
Bristol BS3 1EN
Helpline: 0845 123 2304
Nationwide organisation of and for bereaved parents offering friendship and understanding to other bereaved parents.

CRUSE — Bereavement Care
3 Rutland Square
Edinburgh EH1 2AS
Tel: 0131 229 6275
Fax: 0131 229 9355
email: edinburgh@crusescotland.org.uk
Help, support and counselling for bereaved people.

Foundation for the Study of Infant Deaths (FSID)
Artillery House
11-19 Artillery Row
London SW1P 1RT
Tel: 020 7222 8001
Helpline: 020 7233 2090
Fax: 020 7222 8002
email: fsid@sids.org.uk
www.sids.org.uk/fsid/
Personal support and information for parents who have lost a child through cot death. 24-hour helpline. Runs Care of Next Infant (CONI) programme, providing support and advice for families bereaved by cot death with subsequent children.

Scottish Cot Death Trust
Royal Hospital for Sick Children
Yorkhill
Glasgow G3 8SJ
Tel: 0141 357 3946
Fax: 0141 334 1376
email: h.brooke@clinmed.gla.ac.uk
www.sidscotland.org.uk
Support and information for parents bereaved by sudden infant death. Puts parents in touch with local support groups of other bereaved parents.

Stillbirth and Neonatal Death Society (SANDS)
28 Portland Place
London W1B 1LY
Helpline: 020 7436 5881 (weekdays)
Admin: 020 7436 7940
Fax: 020 7436 3715
email: support@uk-sands.org
www.uk-sands.org
Information and a national network of support groups for bereaved parents.

MENTAL HEALTH

Association for Postnatal Illness (APNI)
145 Dawes Road
Fulham
London SW6 7EB
Tel: 020 7386 0868
Fax: 020 7386 8885
email: info@apni.org
www.apni.org
Network of telephone and postal volunteers who have suffered from postnatal illness and offer information, support and encouragement on a one-to-one basis.

Meet A Mum Association (MAMA)
7 Southcourt Road
Linslade
Leighton Buzzard
Bedfordshire LU7 2QF
Tel: 0845 120 6162
Helpline: 0845 120 3746
email: meet-a-mum.assoc@blueyonder.co.uk
www.mama.co.uk
Offers information and support to mothers suffering postnatal illness. Helps mothers and mothers-to-be who are isolated and lonely by putting them in touch with others for friendship and support.

Scottish Association for Mental Health (SAMH)
Cumbrae House
15 Carlton Court
Glasgow G5 9JP
Tel: 0141 568 7000
Fax: 0141 568 7001
email: enquire@samh.org.uk
www.samh.org.uk
Offers an information service, campaigning and training on mental health issues and deals with any queries on the subject of mental health, and legal and benefits services.

PARENT SUPPORT

BLISS
Tel: 0870 770 0337
Fax: 0870 770 0338
email: information@bliss.org.uk
www.bliss.org.uk
Provides education, resources and support for parents and carers of babies who are, or have been, in special care.

Cry-sis
BM CRY-SIS
London WC1N 3XX
Helpline: 020 7404 5011
email: info@cry-sis.org.uk
Self-help and support for families with excessively crying, sleepless and demanding children via national helpline. Also by post — please enclose SAE.

Gingerbread Scotland
1014 Argyle Street
Glasgow G3 8LX
Tel: 0141 576 5085
Local groups offer mutual support, friendship, information, advice and practical help to one parent families. Welcomes pregnant women.

Home-Start
2 Salisbury Road
Leicester LE1 7QR
Tel: 0116 233 9955
Fax: 0116 233 0232
email: info@home-start.org.uk
www.home-start.org.uk
Offers friendly, practical help and emotional support to families who may be experiencing stress. (Must have at least one child under five years old).

One Parent Families Scotland
13 Gayfield Square
Edinburgh EH1 3NX
Tel: 0131 556 3899
Helpline: 0800 018 5026
Fax: 0131 557 7899
email: info@opfs.org.uk
www.opfs.org.uk
Helps pregnant women, parents bringing up children alone and non-custodial parents. Offers information on welfare rights, housing, childcare, sources of financial help, education and self-help groups.

One Plus — One Parent Families
55 Renfrew Street
Glasgow G2 3BD
Tel: 0141 333 1450
Fax: 0141 3331399
email: enquiries@oneplus.org
www.oneplus.org
Independent organisation for one parent families
offering information, advice and counselling for
individuals and groups of lone parents and their
children. Campaigns to achieve equality of opportunities for
lone parents whether single, widowed, divorced or separated
and regardless of sex, sexuality, race, colour or religion.
Managed by lone parents themselves.

Twins and Multiple Births Association (TAMBA)
2 The Willows
Gardener Road
Guildford, Surrey GU1 4PJ
Tel: 0870 770 3305
Helpline: 0800 138 0509 (evenings)
Fax: 0870 770 3303
email: enquiries@tamba.org.uk
www.tamba.org.uk
Aims to provide information and mutual support
networks for families of twins, triplets and more,
highlighting their unique needs to all involved
in their care.

PREGNANCY & MATERNITY SERVICES

AIMS (Association for Improvements in the Maternity Service)
40 Leamington Terrace
Edinburgh EH10 4JL
Tel: 0131 229 6259
Helpline: 0870 765 1433
www.aims.org.uk
Voluntary pressure group offering support and information
about parents' rights, complaints procedures and choices
within maternity care, including home birth.

Birth Resource Centre Edinburgh
40 Leamington Terrace
Edinburgh EH10 4JL
Tel: 0131 229 3667
email: info@birthresourcecentre.org.uk
www.birthresourcecentre.org.uk
Practical and emotional support for all women and their
families: antenatal and postnatal classes focusing on
movement and relaxation, one-to-one support, sharing
experiences, information, advocacy and child-centred activities
in a warm and welcoming environment.

Lothian Homebirth Support Group
Tel: 0131 478 0659
Provides support and advice for women trying to arrange a
homebirth. Telephone for help and advice.

Maternity Alliance
Third Floor West
2-6 Northburgh Street, London EC1V 0AY
Tel: 020 7490 7639
Information Line: 020 7490 7638
Fax: 020 7014 1350
email: info@maternityalliance.org.uk
www.maternityalliance.org.uk
Campaigns for improvements in rights and services
for mothers, fathers and babies. Provides advice
on healthcare, benefits and employment rights and
an information service for parents and professionals.

Scottish Independent Midwives
9 Cordiner Street (postal only)
Glasgow G44 4TY
Tel: 0141 579 8404
Telephone advice to women who wish to have another
opinion about aspects of their care.

PREGNANCY PROBLEMS

Action on Pre-eclampsia (APEC)
84-88 Pinner Road
Harrow, Middlesex HA1 4HZ
Helpline: 020 8427 4217
Fax: 020 8424 0653
email: info@apec.org.uk
www.apec.org.uk
Charity providing support and information for sufferers
of pre-eclampsia.

Antenatal Results and Choices (ARC)
73-75 Charlotte Street
London W1T 4PN
Helpline: 020 7631 0285
Fax: 020 7631 0280
email: info@arc-uk.org
www.arc-uk.org
Offers support and information to women and couples who
have had a diagnosis of abnormality in their unborn baby, and
provides continued support to those parents who have a
termination of pregnancy.

The Chartered Association Physiotherapy
14 Bedford Row
London WC1R 4ED
Tel: 020 7306 6666
Fax: 020 7306 6611
email: enquiries@csp.org.uk
www.csp.org.uk
Information regarding the role and function of a
chartered physiotherapist, including how to get in
touch with local private practitioners.

Miscarriage Association
c/o Clayton Hospital
Northgate
Wakefield WF1 3JS
Tel: 01924 200799
Fax: 01924 298834
email: info@miscarriageassociation.org.uk
www.miscarriageassociation.org.uk
Information, advice and support for women who have had, or
who are having, a miscarriage.

Obstetric Cholestasis Support Group
4 Shenstone Close
Four Oaks
Sutton Coldfield
Birmingham B74 4XB
Tel: 0121 353 0699
email: jennychambersoc@aol.com
Support and information.

SCIM (Scottish Care and Information on Miscarriage)
41 Merryland Street
Glasgow G51 2QG
Tel: 0141 445 3727
Fax: 0141 445 0119
email: scim@scim.fsworld.co.uk
www.connectedscotland.org.uk/scimnet
Counselling service for women who have lost babies through
miscarriage, support for future pregnancy and planning
pregnancy following loss. Offers individual appointments and
online support group.

RIGHTS & BENEFITS

ACAS (Advisory, Concilliation and Arbitration Service)
151 West George Street
Glasgow G2 7JL
Tel: 0141 248 1400
Public enquiry service: 0845 747 4747
www.acas.org.uk
Provides advice on time off for antenatal care and on
matters such as unfair dismissal. For your local library or
Citizens' Advice Bureau.

Benefit Enquiry Line
0800 88 22 00
Textphone: 0800 24 33 55
Confidential telephone advice and information
service, for people with disabilities, their carers and
representatives. Offers general advice information
about social security benefits and how to claim them.

Child Benefit Office
P.O. Box 1
Newcastle Upon Tyne NE88 1AA
Tel: 0845 302 1444
email: child.benefit@ir.gsi.gov.uk
www.inlandrevenue.gov.uk/
childbenefit/eligible.htm
Offers advice and information about Child Benefits, One
Parent Benefit and Guardian's Allowance.

Child Support Agency
P.O. Box 55
Pedmore House
Brierley Hill
West Midlands DY5 1YL
Tel: 08457 133 133
Minicom: 08457 138 924
www.csa.gov.uk
Government agency which assesses and collects child
maintenance in Great Britain.

Citizen's Advice Bureaux (CABs)
Ask at your local library or look in your phone book under
'Counselling and Advice'.

Commission for Racial Equality
The Tun
12 Jackson's Entry (Off Holyrood Road)
Edinburgh EH8 8PJ
Tel: 0131 524 2000
Fax: 0131 524 2001
email: scotland@cre.gov.uk
www.cre.gov.uk
Works for the elimination of unlawful racial
discrimination and the promotion of equal
opportunities and good race relations.

Edinburgh Disability Benefits Centre (DBC)
Argyle House
3 Lady Lawson Street
Edinburgh EH3 0XY
Tel: 0131 229 9191
Fax: 0131 222 5231
Textphone: 0845 722 4433
www.dss.gov.uk/ba
Information and advice on Attendance Allowance
and Disability Living Allowance. Deals with all areas
in Scotland except Strathclyde (see Glasgow DBC).

Equal Opportunities Commission
St Stevens House, 279 Bath Street
Glasgow G2 4JL
Tel: 0845 601 5901
email: Scotland@eoc.org.uk
www.eoc.org.uk
Information and advice on issues of discrimination
and equal opportunities.

Glasgow Disability Benefits Centre
Corunna House, 29 Cadogan Street
Glasgow G2 7BN
Tel: 0141 249 3500
Information and advice on Attendance Allowance and
Disability Living Allowance. Covers Strathclyde.

Social Security, Department of
For general advice on all social security benefits, child support,
pensions and National Insurance, including maternity benefits
and income support. Telephone, write or call into your local
social security office.

Social Services and Welfare Organisations
For information on topics including benefits, housing, financial
difficulties, employment, relationship
problems, childcare and useful organisations. Look up 'Social
Services' in the phone book under the name of your local
authority or ask at your local library.

VEGETARIANISM

Vegetarian Society of the UK Ltd
Parkdale, Dunham Road
Altrincham
Cheshire WA14 4QG
Tel: 0161 925 2000
Fax: 0161 926 9182
email: info@vegsoc.org
www. vegsoc.org
For general information and advice on all aspects of
vegetarianism. Produces a wide range of resources
including booklets on vegetarianism for babies, children and
pregnant women.

Index

A

abdomen
  muscles, separation/split 55, 102
  palpation 24, 36, 40
abortion *see* miscarriage
abuse, child, contacts 151
accident prevention *see* safety
Additional Maternity Leave 57
adoption 151
aerobics 11
AFP 35, 41, 43
afterpains 102
AIDS 39, 154
Alb (albumin) 35
alcohol
  breastfeeding and 93
  pregnancy and 8
  sources of help 151
allergy, peanut 14, 93, 136
alphafetoprotein (AFP) 35, 41, 43
amniocentesis 41, 43
amniotic sac (bag of waters;
  membranes) 19
  breaking/rupturing 70-1
    artificial 75
  delivery 82
  fluid in (=waters) 35
anaemia 54
anaesthesia
  in Caesarean section 86
  epidural *see* epidural anaesthesia
analgesia 50-1
animals, contact with 14
antenatal appointments/care
  28, 29, 34-43, 56
  asking questions 43
  time-off to attend 23
  words used by staff 35-6
antenatal (parentcraft) classes
  29, 64-5
  non-NHS 65
  time-off to attend 23
antibodies *see* immunity
antidepressants 108
Apgar score 83
APH (antepartum haemorrhage/
  bleeding) 18, 35, 54

B

baby (born) 88-150
  appearance at birth 79
  death *see* cot death; miscarriage;
    stillbirth
  development *see* development
  due date 5
  first days 88-90
  greeting your baby 83
  health benefits of breastfeeding
    38, 93
  illness *see* illness
  preparing for 66
  preterm *see* preterm babies
  routine care 110-14
  support services *see* support
baby (unborn) *see* fetus
'baby blues' 103, 107
baby slings 114, 118
backache 28, 31, 53
bathing 66, 110-11
  safety 132
bearing down 77
bed(s) 114, 117
bed-wetting 147

behavioural problems, sources
  of help 151
benefits 23, 57-9
  useful addresses 155
bereavement *see* cot death;
  miscarriage; stillbirth
birth 46-51, 77-81
  choosing where/how 46-51
  difficult, talking about 106
  moment of 78
  preparing for 30-1
  preterm *see* preterm babies
  registering 89
birth plan 48
blastocyst 17
bleeding/haemorrhage
  gums 52
  vaginal
    antepartum 18, 35, 54
    postpartum 83, 102
blood pressure
  high (hypertension)
    35, 36, 39, 55
  low 35
  measurement 39, 56
blood tests 39
'bloom' of pregnancy 10
books 140
bottle feeding 99-101
  breastfeeding after period of 97
  breastfeeding mixed with 38, 97
  making up feeds 101
  phasing out 137
  planning 48
  sweet (sugary) drinks 141
  vitamins drops and 138
bowel movements *see* stools
boy or girl? 45
BR (breech presentation)
  33, 35, 61
bra, maternity 25
Braxton Hicks contractions 33
breast(s), *see also* nipples
  changes after birth 102
  changes in pregnancy 4, 18
  colostrum 27, 29, 92
breast milk
  expressing 29, 66, 97, 98
  iron in 141
  not enough 95
breast pump 66, 98
breastfeeding 38, 91-7
  aids to success 38
  bottle feeding mixed with 38, 97
  Caesarean section and 87
  contraception and 105
  difficulties 95
  drugs and 93, 108
  first/early 38, 83, 84, 91-4
  health benefits 38, 93
  later 94, 96, 97
  planning 48
  preterm baby 29
  stopping (weaning) 99,
    127-8, 137
  support/useful addresses 95, 151
  twins 61
  vitamins drops and 138
breathing
  fetal 32
  in labour 50
breech presentation 33, 35, 61

C

Caesarean section 85-7
  breech presentation and 33
  exercise and 102

supportive organisations 153
  with twins/triplets 60
candidiasis (thrush) 52, 95
car safety 90, 131
  seat belt 90, 131
casein-based formula milk 99
cats 14
centile chart 122
cephalic (ceph/vertex)
  position 35
  twins 61
cereals
  baby 136
  mother 13, 14
cervix
  colour changes 18
  incompetence 68
cheese, soft ripened 14
chemicals, dangerous 23
child abuse, contacts 151
Child Benefit 59
child health clinic 122
childcare, useful addresses
  151-2
cholestasis 55
chorionic gonadotrophin
    see human chorionic
    gonadotrophin
chorionic villus sampling (CVS)
  41, 42
chromosomal disorders 41
claims, making 58
clothes
  baby 66, 113
  maternity 25
colic 118
colostrum 27, 29, 92
communication *see* hearing;
  seeing; talking; touch
companions *see* friends;
  partners
conception 17
constipation 52, 102
consultant-led unit 46
contraception
  breastfeeding and 105
  oral (pill) 105
  useful addresses 153
contractions 71-75
  3rd stage of labour 82, 83
  Braxton Hicks 33
  postpartum 102
  stopping/fading away 71, 75
cord *see* umbilical cord
cot 66, 114, 117
cot death (sudden unexpected
    death) 116
  useful addresses 154
cow's milk/milk products 99, 136
crib 66, 114
crowning 77
crying 118
  illness 150
cups 137
cystic fibrosis (CF) 42, 88
  CF trust 152
cystitis 53
cytomegalovirus 42

D

dairy foods, mother 13
dangers *see* safety
date, due 5
death of baby *see* cot death;
  miscarriage; stillbirth

delivery *see* Caesarean section;
  labour
dentist 141
depression, postnatal 107-9
  useful addresses 154
development/progress 119-50
  before birth 17-34
  after birth 119-50
    assessment 122
    charts 119-20
diabetes 40, 54
  British Diabetic Assoc. 152
diagnostic tests 41, 41-3
  problem detected in 43
diamorphine 51
diet *see* food
dietician 37
diphtheria vaccine 125
disability, useful addresses
  152-3
dislocation of hip, congenital
  88
doctor, family 37
domino birth 46
Doppler ultrasound in labour
  74
double test 41
Down's syndrome 41, 43
  Scottish Down's Syndrome Assoc.
    153
dreaming 63
drugs *see also* specific (types
  of) *drugs*
  breastfeeding and 93, 108
  pregnancy and 8
  sources of help 151
DTaP/IPV/Hib vaccine 125
due date 5

E

eating *see* food
eclampsia 55, 86
ectopic pregnancy 35, 68
egg, implantation 17, 18
electronic fetal monitoring 74
embryo 17, 19
employer's legal obligation 23
engagement of head 32, 35
Entonox 51
epidural anaesthesia 51
  Caesarean section 86
episiotomy 35, 81
equipment (for baby) 114
  bottle feeding 100, 101
  safety 131, 132
exercise(s) 11-12
  pelvic floor 52, 102, 103

F

facial features, fetus 21
family 104
family doctor 37
family planning *see* contraception
fathers *see* partners
fatigue *see* tiredness
feeding *see* food (baby)
feet 10
fetal alcohol syndrome 8
fetus 17-34
  awareness of surroundings 62-3
  death *see* miscarriage; stillbirth

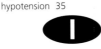